Flu Pandemic

The Complete Story of the Spanish Flu of 1918 and the other
Deadliest Pandemics that changed the course of History

By

Bryan Anderson

CONTENTS

Pandemics History

THE SPANISH FLU

Pandemics History

How Plague, Cholera, Spanish Flu and Other Deadly
Epidemics have Changed the World and its Society

Introduction: The Pandemic

A pandemic (from Greek πν) pan, "all" and δμος, Demos, "individuals") is an epidemic of illness that's spread across a huge area, for example, multiple continents or globally, affecting a considerable number of individuals. An endemic disease using a number of individuals isn't a pandemic. Widespread diseases having a number of individuals like recurrences of flu are excluded as they happen in areas of the planet as opposed to being dispersed. There are quite a few pandemics of diseases like tuberculosis and smallpox. The fatal pandemic listed in history was that the Black Death (also called The Plague), which killed an estimated 75-200 million people in the 14th century. Other noteworthy pandemics include the 1918 flu pandemic (Spanish influenza). Current pandemics comprise HIV/AIDS and COVID-19. An influenza pandemic happens when a new flu virus emerges and spreads around the world, and individuals don't have immunity. Viruses that have caused pandemics originated from animal flu viruses. While other characteristics might be distinct, some facets of flu pandemics can seem similar to the flu. For instance, both seasonal and pandemic flu can cause illnesses in all age classes, and many cases will end in self-limited illness where the individual recovers fully without treatment. But typical seasonal flu causes many of its deaths among the older while other acute cases occur most commonly in people who have various health ailments. By comparison, this H1N1 outbreak caused nearly all of its acute or deadly disorder in younger individuals, those with chronic conditions, in addition to healthy men, and caused several more instances of viral pneumonia than is generally diagnosed with seasonal flu. For both seasonal and pandemic flu, the number of folks who get seriously ill can differ. On the other hand, the effect of seriousness will be greater in pandemics in part due to the much larger amount of men and women of the people who lack preexisting resistance to the new virus. When a sizable part of the populace is infected, even if the percentage of those infected go on to develop acute disease is small, the entire number of acute cases is often very large. For both seasonal and pandemic flu, the levels of action would be anticipated to happen in the flu season interval for a place (from the temperate climate zones, this is ordinarily the wintertime, for instance). However, as was observed with the present H1N1 pandemic, pandemics could have abnormal epidemiological patterns and massive outbreaks may happen in summertime months. Pandemics are conditions of disorder that sharply grow in populations around the planet with illnesses occurring more or less concurrently. While it normally describes infectious diseases, such as plague or flu, it's frequently utilized to refer to additional health ailments, including obesity, cancer, as well as addiction. Pathogen transmission by means of a populace is normally coated by five typical descriptions. An infection is one that stays steady with time, infecting a variety of hosts in a way that is normally well known. The parasite schistosomiasis, as an instance, can result in ailments, but is comprised in amounts that don't change much from year to year within areas. An epidemic refers to a spike in transmissions at a region that is localized. For instance, in 2019 the Democratic Republic of the Congo saw a steep increase in people contracting the Ebola virus from the country's east. While the World Health Organization (WHO) seen it as a public health crisis, its containment supposed it was not an outbreak. Outbreaks across areas are normally considered epidemics. The spread of Ebola across Western Africa between 2016 and 2013 is described with the term epidemic. When the outbreak has turned out to be effective at moving around the entire world in a manner that sustains prevalent, continuing infections, it may be considered a pandemic.

The Next Pandemic

A virus is being closely watched by the entire world Flu H5N1, or "bird flu. " Now it is understood that the virus is deadly, and that people who have caught the virus from poultry that was sick. Scientists fear that at any stage the H5N1 virus may mutate to a form that could pass from humans. "When it adapts into a breed that is infectious among people it will no more be a bird virus. It will grow to be a human flu virus," Epstein tells WebMD. If this strain can pass easily between people, it might turn into a pandemic influenza. "It is not possible to predict if this virus will mutate enough to be readily passable from human to human," Pearson tells WebMD. The following flu pandemic is a certainty. However, the next pandemic may be caused by an entirely different virus. It will not grow from H5N1.

Difference Between An Epidemic Plus Also A Pandemic

Epidemic is any problem which has grown out of control. An outbreak is defined as "an epidemic of an illness that happens over a huge geographic area and impacts an exceptionally large percentage of the populace. " An outbreak is an event where there is a disorder dispersing. By comparison, the expression pandemic relates to spread and can be used to refer to a disorder which affects the world or a nation. While casual usage of outbreaks may not call for these nuances, it is important that you be aware of the differences between both of these conditions (and similar types such as epidemic and endemic) when considering general health information. In an epidemiologic perspective, additionally, conditions like these lead the public health response and stop a disorder.

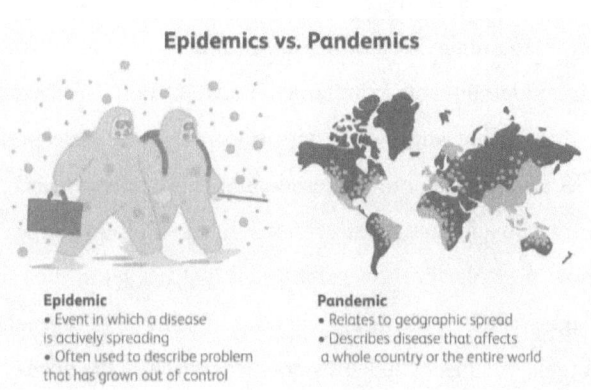

Epidemics vs. Pandemics

Epidemic
• Event in which a disease is actively spreading
• Often used to describe problem that has grown out of control

Pandemic
• Relates to geographic spread
• Describes disease that affects a whole country or the entire world

Common Confusion

While epidemic is utilized to describe things of health (e. g. the opioid catastrophe in the USA has increased to epidemic proportions), it's occasionally used colloquially to explain behavior (There is an outbreak of bursts among preschoolers!) Or behavioral phenomena (like "epidemic hysteria"). They could lead to confusion while the usages aren't inappropriate in the context. Additionally, even if the term is used to identify health difficulties, it might not accurately portray development or the scale of a disorder. Sometimes, conditions like endemic or epidemic might be more suitable. In the others, the outbreak may fall short in describing the problem's scale and be defined as a pandemic.

Epidemic Vs. Pandemic

While the terms might suggest that there's a specific edge in which an event is announced regarding an outbreak, thus the distinction between epidemic, and pandemics blurred. Part of the reason behind this is that some disorders become more widespread or deadly as time passes, but some become less, forcing the CDC to frequently adjust its statistical versions. Epidemiologists are careful about how they clarify a disorder event that it's set in the context that is right. While a disorder that's out of control is suggested by an outbreak, events called clusters to guarantee an occasion of concern. The CDC admits that specific conditions can exude anxiety that is undue. 1 instance is that the Zika epidemic of 2016, which triggered an alarm when disease happened in six individuals in Texas and 218 people in Florida. The other 46 were infected by lab transmission or sexual, and a single individual became infected by contact. Despite HIV, outbreak has replaced the expression pandemic given the distribution of Treatment and rates in certain regions that were formerly hyper-prevalent. On the flip side, as flu gets more virulent year annually, public health officials may generally refer to the seasonal outbreaks as pandemics, especially awarded the 2009 H1N1 outbreak in the USA where over 60 million Americans were impacted, leading to 274,304 hospitalizations and 12,469 deaths. This isn't to imply that pandemics are approached as a more constrained outbreak. When it has the capability to extend beyond its own boundaries, such as can happen with the Ebola 35, on the reverse side, an epidemic might be treated than a pandemic. Feelings of doubt, depression, anxiety, and dread are normal during pandemics. Becoming proactive about your health can help keep both your body and mind stronger. Learn about the very best treatment alternatives.

Phases Of A Pandemic

While there are ways to assess and classify an illness occasion, the actual staging of an outbreak (basically the outline regarding if the spread of illness is acute enough to take certain activities) can vary dependent on the pathogenesis (pathway) of a disorder and many other epidemiological aspects. The 1 staging model utilized to guide the public health response especially involves influenza (the flu). Back in 1999, the World Health Organization (WHO) published the very first flu pandemic preparedness plan where it summarized the proper answer based on six obviously summarized stages. The goal of the strategy was supposed to coordinate the worldwide response by offering states a blueprint where to draw their own national plans based on available funds. Its pandemic flu plan was released by America. The standard model may be implemented with variants such as the Zika virus, malaria, as well as tuberculosis, into epidemics. Phases 1 through 3 are intended to aid public health officials in understanding now is the time to come up with action plans and the resources to react to an impending hazard. The WHO revised the stages to distinguish between response and preparedness. The strategy was meant to deal with flu pandemics, awarded their high mutation rate, and the ability of the virus.

Former WHO Stages of Pandemic

- **Stage 1** is the interval during which no creature viruses have been reported to cause disease in people.
- **Stage 2** is the initial amount of danger wherein a virus has been verified to have jumped from an animal to people.
- **Stage 3** is when sporadic cases or tiny clusters of illness are verified, but human-to-human transmission has not occurred or has been deemed unlikely to sustain an epidemic.
- **Stage 4** is the stage where both human-to-humans and human-animal virus has generated a community-wide

20

outbreak.

- **Stage 5** is when human-to-human transmission of this virus has resulted in the spread of illness to two nations.
- **Stage 6** is the stage where the disorder has announced a pandemic, which spread to at least another nation.

The timeframe for every phase can vary considerably, ranging from months to decades. Not all will advance to stage 6. Some viruses may weaken or even revert.

Chapter 1: Cholera (1817-1923)

Cholera is an acute infectious disease brought on by a Bacterium, Vibrio cholera (V. cholerae), which normally ends in a painless, watery diarrhea in people. Some people create dehydration and have copious quantities of nausea, which may cause death. Many of us who get the disorder ingest the organisms through food or water resources infected with V. cholerae. Though symptoms can be mild, a few healthy men and women will create diarrhea in about a couple of times. Disease demands immediate medical attention. Hydration (generally by IV using a rehydration solution for it's very sick) of the individual, and antibiotics in certain people, is the secret to surviving the acute life-threatening type of the disease. Subtypes of V. cholerae that might result in acute cases comprise 01 and 0139. The World Health Organization (WHO) includes maps of present and previous regions with cholera outbreaks (see WHO benchmark). It's estimated that roughly 1. 4 million to 4. 3 million individuals are infected globally annually, with roughly 28,000-142,000 deaths each year. Just about 1 in 10 people create symptoms and the signs. Outbreaks of cholera in 2015-2016 comprise South Sudan, United Republic of Tanzania, and Kenya, with over 216 deaths. Lately, 121 individuals diagnosed with cholera in Iraq, their initial outbreak since 2012, and in Cuba, the initial epidemic in over 130 decades. The expression cholera has a very long history (see history section under) and has been delegated to other ailments. For instance, poultry or fowl cholera is a disorder that could kill other parasitic species and cows using a symptom of nausea. On the other hand, the broker in fowl is a bacterium, Pasteurellamultocida. In the same way, pig cholera (also termed hog or swine cholera) may cause rapid death (in around 15 times) in hens with symptoms of fever, skin lesions, as well as seizures. This disorder is due to a pestivirus termed CSFV (classical swine fever virus). The language may be confusing, although none of those animal diseases are linked to cholera.

As a highly contagious disease, cholera spreads quite reverently within and between states and areas. In accordance with the WHO, there are 100,000-200,000 deaths each year and still an estimated 3-5 million cases. Outbreaks change in intensity: prevalence rates generally vary from under 0. 1% to approximately 0. 4%, case fatality rates vary from 0. 5% to 10 percent and epidemics continue from a few weeks to more than 1 year. The disorder is transmitted through the ingestion of polluted water and food, and consequently, it is more widespread in developing nations where access to water is constrained. Approximately 75 percent of the populace could be infected but show no indication of illness, leading to the spreading of the disease whenever folks travel between areas. Immediate treatment combined with access to sanitation and safe water and health instruction can limit the disease's effect. The case fatality rate for those infected is 1 percent, but this may grow when origin is ineffective or if no treatment is administered. The WHO reports a case fatality rate of 6 percent at the start of the 2009 outbreak. Consequently, access to Treatment and the inherent water infrastructure and schooling levels ascertain both the disease and death rates existing inside a nation, and if they are rising due to the circumstances. Thus, the societal and financial costs of a cholera outbreak can be anticipated. Within this report, the historic benchmarks of former cholera epidemics have been described. As mentioned from the literature and data recorded by the International Vaccine Institute (IVI), we estimate that the financial effect of a cholera epidemic in Bangladesh and Mozambique. We utilize the Oxford Economics model to catch the principal classes, such as supply and demand effects. Considering that Oxford Economics' version doesn't include Bangladesh and Mozambique, we scale the shocks in line with Bangladesh and Mozambique's characteristics and utilize versions for India and South Africa. India and South Africa share many similar economic characteristics that indicate the transmission of the shock through the market is very likely to be like what could occur in Bangladesh and Mozambique.

The History Of Cholera

Humans for centuries have been impacted due to this disorder. Reports of disorder have been observed in India as near the beginning as 1000 AD. Cholera is a name stemmed from Greek khole (disease from bile) and afterward from the 14th century into colere (French) and choler (English). From the 17th century was a phrase used to refer to a serious disease Nausea and nausea. There were outbreaks and a few were noted in ancient writings. England had a few; the most celebrated being in 1854, the 19th century, when Dr. John Snow did a Timeless research in London that revealed a principal source of the disorder (leading to roughly 500 deaths in 10 times) came from a minimum of one of the significant water resources for London residents termed the "Broad Street pump." The pump is present as a milestone in London. Although the cause was not discovered by Dr. Snow of cholera, he'd reveal the disease can be spread and the way to prevent a neighborhood outbreak. This was the start of contemporary studies. The final reference indicates the map Dr. Snow utilized to recognize the pump website. V. cholerae was isolated as the reason for cholera from Filippo Pacini in 1854, but his discovery wasn't widely understood until Robert Koch (who discovered the cause of tuberculosis), functioning independently 30 decades afterward, publicized the knowledge and the way of combating with the illness. The foundation of cholera recaps itself. The U. S. National Library of Medicine houses first records about multiple cholera outbreaks from the U. S. in the 1820s into the 1900s, together with the Last epidemic in 1910-1911. There were seven Cholera pandemics (global outbreaks). The 7 pandemic of cholera begin in 1961 and continued until 1975; the occasional is thought by a few investigators. Outbreaks (up to the current time) represent fires of this seventh pandemic. Cholera riots happened in Russia and England (1831), and in Germany (1893) if the people rebelled against rigorous authorities' isolation (quarantines) and burial principles. In Zimbabwe, cholera riots broke out in 2008 as police attempted to disperse individuals who were and also strove to draw money protesting due to the collapse of the health system, which started with a cholera outbreak. Similar but less violent protests have happened when Typhoid fever, yellow fever, and tuberculosis quarantines are enforced by health authorities. Outbreaks persist in the 21st century, with outbreaks in India, Iran, Vietnam, and many African nations over the past 10 decades. Some outbreaks happened in Nigeria and Haiti and, in 2010-2011, South Sudan, Tanzania, Iraq, Kenya, Cuba, and in Yemen. Considering that in 2017-2018, the WHO recorded instances of Cholera with 2,267 related deaths in Yemen. Is cholera background repeating itself? The solution could be traced back to the research of Dr. Snow, which revealed a supply (water-borne or sometimes food) infected with V. cholerae may rapidly and easily transmit the germs. Until water and food is available to most people, it is very likely that Cholera outbreaks will continue to take place.

Origins Of Cholera

It is unclear when men and women were influenced by cholera. Ancient texts in India (from Sushruta Samhita from the 5th century B. C.) and Greece (Hippocrates in the 4th century B. C. and Aretaeus of Cappadocia from the 1st century A. D.) describe isolated instances of cholera-like ailments. Among the earliest detailed reports of cholera outbreak comes from Gaspar Correa-- Portuguese historian and writer of Legendary India--that described an epidemic in the spring of 1543 of a disorder from the Ganges Delta, which can be found in the southwest Asia region of Bangladesh and India. The regional people called the disorder "moryxy," and it allegedly killed victims in seven hours of developing symptoms and had a fatality rate so large that sailors

26

fought to bury all the dead. Various reports of India along the west coast were filed from observers.

The First Cholera Pandemic

The cholera pandemic emerged from the Ganges Delta. Having an epidemic in Jessore, India, in 1817, originating from rice that was polluted. The disease spread through the Majority of India Myanmar Modern – day Sri Lanka -- by travel along trade routes Europeans. By 1820, cholera had spread into Thailand, Indonesia (murdering 100,000 individuals around the island of Java independently), and the Philippines. From Thailand, the disease made its way to Japan in 1822 and China from 1820 by means of individuals on boats. Additionally, it spread beyond Asia. In British, 1821 Cholera was attracted by soldiers traveling from India to Oman and brought cholera to the Persian Gulf. The disease made its way to land Turkey, Southern Russia, and Syria. The pandemic died out 6 years after it began, likely thanks to a severe winter in 1823–1824, which may have killed the bacteria living in water supplies.

1846--1860 Cholera Pandemic

The next cholera pandemic (1846-60) was the third largest important outbreak of cholera originating in the nineteenth century, which reached far in India and continued until 1863 (it could have begun as early as 1837). In Russia, more than one million people died of cholera. Over 10,000 lives, the outbreak in London claimed Back in 1853 -- 54, and also there were 23,000 deaths for all of Great Britain. This pandemic was believed to have the deaths of these epidemics. It had deaths among inhabitants in Africa, Europe, Asia, and North America. In the season of 1854, it was believed that 23,000 people died in Great Britain. That year, the British physician John Snow, who was working in a poor area of London, identified contaminated water as the means of transmission of the disease. He had mapped the instances of cholera in London at the Soho area, and also noticed that a bunch of cases close to a water pump. To test his theory, officials persuaded to remove the pump handle, and also the number of cholera cases in the region diminished. His breakthrough helped bring the outbreak under control. Snow was a member of London, formed in reaction. He's considered one of the fathers of epidemiology.

1899--1923 Cholera Pandemic

The cholera pandemic had a small impact in Europe due to improvements in public health; however, the Ottoman Empire, as well as important cities was hard hit by cholera deaths. More than 500,000 people died of cholera from 1900 to 1925, which was a period of disruption due to warfare and revolution in Russia. The 1902-1904 cholera outbreak claimed 200,000 lives from the Philippines, likePrime Minister Apolinario Mabini and their hero. Cholera broke out 27 times during the hajj at Mecca from the 19th century to 1930. The sixth pandemic killed more than 800,000 in India. The outbreak in the USA was in 1910-1911, once individuals were brought by the steamship Moltke from Naples. Vigilant health authorities circulated the contaminated on Swinburne Island in quarantine. Eleven people died, such as a health care worker at the hospital around the island. Since travelers and immigrants carried cholera from locales, the disorder became correlated with outsiders in every single society. The Italians blamed the Jews and gypsies, the British that had been in India detained the "filthy natives," and also the Americans believed the disease came from the Philippines.

Cholera Infects Europe And The Americas

The cholera pandemic started around 1829. Like the one that came before it, the next pandemic is supposed to have originated in India and spread across military and trade routes to Eastern and Central Asia and the Middle East. By the fall of 1830, it had been forced by cholera. The spread of this disease slowed through the winter months, but picked up again in the spring of 1831, attaining Poland and Finland. It passed to Germany and Hungary. The disorder then spread across Europe, such as hitting Great Britain for the first time through the interface of Sunderland in late 1831 and London in the spring of 1832. Britain enacted activities to help curb the spread of this disease, such as executing quarantines and establishing boards of health. Nevertheless, the people became gripped with fear of this illness and distrust of authority figures. Unbalanced media reporting directed people to believe more victims perished in the hospital compared to their houses, and the people began to feel that sufferers taken to hospitals had been murdered by physicians for anatomical dissection, a result they called "Burking. " This panic resulted in many "cholera riots" in Liverpool. Cholera had made it. In June of the year, Quebec watched 1,000 deaths in the illness, which rapidly spread across the St. Lawrence River and its tributaries. Cholera imported in the USA, appearing at Philadelphia and New York. Across the nation, it might spread during the next few years. It attained Latin America, such as Cuba and Mexico. The pandemic reemerged throughout nations for almost two years before it subsided around 1851 and would perish.

What Are The Signs And Cholera Symptoms?

Cholera-related disease's signs and symptoms are watery diarrhea which often includes flecks of whitish material (mucus along with a few gastrointestinal liner epithelial cells which are about the size of bits of rice.) The nausea is known as "rice-water stool" and smells "fishy. " Though a lot of bacterial infections can lead to diarrhea, the quantity of nausea with cholera may be substantial; large levels of diarrheal fluid, for example 250 cc per kg roughly 10 to 18 liters over 24 hours to get a 154-pound grownup, can happen. Individuals may go on to create one or more of these signs and symptoms:

- Watery diarrhea (occasionally in Massive volumes)

- Rice-water stools
- Fishy odor to stools
- Vomiting
- Quick heart rate
- Loss of skin elasticity (washer girl palms sign;
- Dry mucous membranes (dry mouth)
- Low blood pressure
- Thirst
- Muscle cramps (leg cramps, for example)
- Restlessness or irritability (particularly in children)
- Unusual sleepiness or fatigue

Other symptoms that may occur, particularly with more severe illness, include the following:

- Abdominal pain (cramps)
- Rectal pain
- Fever
- Severe vomiting
- Dehydration
- Low or no urine output
- Weight reduction
- Seizures
- Shock
- Death

Those infected need hydration to stop these symptoms from

continuing because symptoms and these signs suggest that the individual has become or is about to develop acute cholera. Individuals with severe cholera (roughly 5%-10% of formerly healthy individuals; greater if people are jeopardized by poor nutrition or contain a higher proportion of very young or older people) can create severe dehydration, resulting in severe renal failure, acute electrolyte imbalances (especially potassium and sodium), and coma. This dehydration may cause death and shock if untreated. Severe dehydration may happen four to eight hours end to a couple of days in men and women that are undertreated or untreated. Outbreaks in underdeveloped nations, where little or no treatment is available, the mortality (death) rate is often as large as 50%-60%.

Approximately 80 percent who do not develop the disease resolves by itself and cholera symptoms. And of 20 percentage come down with symptoms, including nausea and leg cramps. These indicators may lead to dehydration, septic shock, and even death in a matter of just a couple of hours. People who contract non-01 or even non-1039 V. cholerae may also acquire a diarrheal disorder, but it's not more intense than real cholera. Now, cholera is medicated via replacement and antibiotics. Even though they offer approximately 65% resistance, in accordance with WHO, cholera vaccines can be found.

What Causes Cholera, And How Can Cholera Spread?

Cholera is caused by the bacterium vibrio cholera. This infection is gram stain-negative, comma-shaped, also contains a flagellum (a long, tapering, casting component) to get motility and pili (hairlike structures) used to attach tissue. Even though there are numerous V. cholerae serotypes that may create cholera symptoms, the O bands O1 and O139, which also create a poison, cause the most acute signs of cholera. O groups contain distinct constructions on the face of germs, which are distinguished from methods. The poison produced by those V. cholerae serotypes is an enterotoxin consisting of 2 subunits, A and B; the genetic in sequence for the production of the subunits is encoded on plasmids (genetic elements different from the bacterial chromosome). Additionally, a different plasmid type encodes for a pilus (a hollow hair like structure which encourages bacterial attachment to individual cells and ease the movement of poison from V. cholerae into individual cells). The enterotoxin induces human cells to extract water and electrolytes in the body (primarily the higher gastrointestinal tract -- little intestine) and inflate it into the intestinal lumen in which the fluid and electrolytes are excreted as diarrheal liquid. The enterotoxin is very similar to toxin generated by germs, which cause diphtheria because both bacterial forms secret the toxins in their surrounding environment in which the poison subsequently enters the individual cells. The bacteria are transmitted by drinking water. However, the bacteria may be consumed in food, particularly seafood, such as oysters.

What Are Risk Factors For Cholera

Everyone who eats or drinks food that has not been treated to remove V. cholerae (fluids will need to be chemically treated, boiled, or pasteurized, and foods will need to be cooked and cleaned), particularly in regions of the world where cholera exists, is at risk for cholera. Outbreaks occur when there are other motives or disasters for a reduction of individual waste disposal along with the shortage of fluids and foods for individuals. Haiti, a nation that hadn't seen a cholera epidemic in more than 50 decades, had such conditions grow in 2010 when a huge earthquake ruined sanitary facilities and water and food treatment centers for several Haitians. Post-earthquake, V. cholera bacteria finally contaminated primary water resources, leading to over 530,000 individuals diagnosed with cholera that led to over 7,000 deaths. This cholera outbreak spread to the neighbor of Haiti. The Vibrio cholerae strain was directly linked to a strain set up in Nepal and contributed some people to blame Nepalese troops (United Nations help troops) that aided with the earthquake catastrophe since the origin of this Haiti cholera outbreak. In 2010, the United Nations Secretary-General,' Ban Ki-moon, apologized for its outbreak that initially developed near a U. N. base. In third-world nations, appetite can direct individuals to accidentally eat polluted food and/or drink polluted water, thus increasing the danger of cholera to infect malnourished populations. There's some evidence that V. cholerae could live in saltwater and also have already been isolated from shellfish; eating raw shellfish is regarded as a risk factor for cholera, particularly in underdeveloped nations and sometimes even in developed nations. A couple of men and women are diagnosed with cholera each year from the U. S. Many of those people diagnosed are travelers that have been exposed to cholera beyond the nation, but sometimes, isolated instances are traced to contaminated seafood, normally from countries that border the Gulf of Mexico. Some people are at greater risk to become infected than others. Individuals that are immune-compromised or malnourished are far more inclined to get the illness. Kids ages 2-4 appear more vulnerable according to some researchers. Additionally, scientists have noted that individuals with blood type O are twice as likely to come up with cholera others. The cause of this particular blood type isn't totally recognized. People along with achlorhydria (reduced acid secretion in the gut) and individuals taking medications to decrease stomach acid (H2 blockers and many others) are more likely to come up with cholera because stomach acid kills various kinds of bacteria, such as V. cholerae.

The Incubation Period For Cholera

The incubation period (time interval from exposure to the germs into the growth of symptoms) can differ from a couple of hours (approximately six to 12 hours) to five times, with the normal incubation period being about two to three times. Approximately six to 12 hours is regarded as an extremely quick incubation period and might imply that rapid/immediate intervention is necessary for recovery.

The Infectious Time For Cholera

The period for cholera starts organisms are excreted in the stool. This may last for approximately seven to 14 days and may happen to the bacteria. Some people that are asymptomatic (infected but not having symptoms) may even excrete infectious organisms for approximately seven to 14 days.

The Remedy For Cholera

The CDC (and virtually every medical bureau) urges rehydration with ORS (oral rehydration salts) fluids as the most important remedy for cholera. ORS fluids can be found in prepackaged container-available globally, and comprise of sugar and electrolytes. The CDC follows the plan urbanized by the WHO (World Health Organization) as follows:

WHO Fluid Replacement or Treatment Recommendations (as per the CDC)

Patient condition	Treatment	Treatment volume guidelines; age and weight
No dehydration	Oral rehydration salts (ORS)	Children < 2 years: 50 mL-100 mL, up to 500 mL/day Children 2-9 years: 100 mL-200 mL, up to 1,000 mL/day Patients > 9 years: As much as wanted, to 2,000 mL/day
Some dehydration	Oral rehydration salts (amount in first four hours)	Infants < 4 mos (< 5 kg): 200-400 mL Infants 4 mos-11 mos (5 kg-7.9 kg): 400-600 mL Children 1 yr-2 yrs (8 kg-10.9 kg): 600-800 mL Children 2 yrs-4 yrs (11 kg-15.9 kg): 800-1,200 mL Children 5 yrs-14 yrs (16 kg-29.9 kg): 1,200-2,200 mL Patients > 14 yrs (30 kg or more): 2,200-4,000 mL
Severe dehydration	IV drips of Ringer Lactate or, if not available, normal saline and oral rehydration salts as outlined above	Age < 12 months: 30 mL/kg within one hour*, then 70 mL/kg over five hours Age > 1 year: 30 mL/kg within 30 min*, then 70 mL/kg over two and a half hours

* Recap once if radial pulse is even very feeble or not detectable

- Reassess the patient a couple of hours and keep hydrating. If hydration isn't improving, give the IV drip more quickly. 200 mL/kg or more could be required during the initial 24 hours of Treatment.
- Following six hours (infants) or 3 hours (elderly patients), perform a complete reassessment. Switch to ORS alternative if hydration is enhanced and the patient can consume.

Generally, antibiotics are reserved for more severe cholera infections; they work to decrease fluid rehydration amounts and might speed recovery. Though great microbiological principles dictate that it's ideal to treat a patient using antibiotics, which are proven to be effective from the infecting bacteria, this can take a long time a time to achieve through a first outbreak (however it should be tried); nonetheless, acute infections have been doctored with tetracycline (Sumycin), doxycycline (Vibramycin, Oracea, Adoxa, Atridox(and many others), furazolidone (Furoxone), erythromycin (E-Mycin, Eryc, Ery-Tab, PCE, Pediazole, Ilosone), or ciprofloxacin (Cipro, CiproXR, ProQuinXR) in conjunction with the next antibiotics along with IV hydration and electrolytes:

- Tetracycline (Sumycin)
- Doxycycline (Vibramycin, Oracea, Adoxa, Atridox, along with many others)
- Furazolidone (Furoxone)
- Erythromycin (E-Mycin, Eryc, Ery-Tab, PCE, Pediazole, Ilosone)
- Azithromycin (Zithromax)
- Sulfamethoxazole/trimethoprim (Bactrim, Septra)
- Ampicillin
- Ciprofloxacin (Cipro, CiproXR, ProQuinXR)
- Norfloxacin (Noroxin)

Many antibiotics have been recorded due to widespread antibiotic resistance, such as vibrio breeds, antibiotic susceptibility testing is recommended so the antibiotic is preferred. Additionally, quinolones (by way of instance, ciprofloxacin, norfloxacin) shouldn't be utilized in children if other antibiotics may be effective due to potential musculoskeletal adverse results.

Is It Feasible To Prevent Cholera? Are Cholera Vaccines Out There?

Yes, numerous techniques can prevent cholera. Developed nations possess an almost zero prevalence of cholera since they have widespread water-treatment plants, food-preparation centers that normally practice sanitary protocols, and the majority of people have access to bathrooms and hand-washing facilities. They've prevented disease outbreaks, such as cholera, though these countries might have openings or lapses within these methods. People can stop or decrease the chance of getting cholera by thorough hand washing, avoiding people and areas with cholera, drinking water or similar secure fluids, and eating cleaned and well-cooked food. Moreover, there are vaccines available that could help prevent cholera, even though they're unavailable from the U. S. , and their efficacy ranges from 50%-90%, based upon the research reported. Since vaccines haven't been shown to be powerful, the vaccines are cholera vaccines. 2 vaccines (Shanchol and Dukoral) are collected of killed V. cholera bacteria and do not include the enterotoxin B subunit. But one report indicates that Shanchol is roughly 65% successful over five decades, both provide protection for just about two decades. Both sexes are generally given in 2 doses. Sad to say, accessibility has been limited by the vaccines; their usage is for individuals going together with the potential to regions of outbreaks. Some investigators suggest this vaccine accessibility that is restricted ought to be changed and mention data that restrict outbreaks may be helped by medication once they've begun. Research is continuing; a research study in Haiti will attempt to learn whether a two-dose vaccine in people will suffice. You will find over 30 universities exploring this disease (cholera's epidemiology, pathology, immunology, vaccine manufacturing, along with other issues) now globally. In 2015, roughly 2 million doses of oral cholera vaccine were sent to several outbreak regions, and currently available data indicates there was a substantial decrease in transmission of endemic cholera; the analysis will be concluded it 2018. In June 2016, the U. S. FDA (Food and Drug management) accepted the early vaccination available from the United States to reduce cholera. The vaccine is known as Vaxchora and is fabricated by PaxVax Bermuda LTD. It may be utilized in adult's age 18-64 that are currently traveling to regions of earth. The vaccine is an attenuated (weakened) amount of V. choleraeserogroup 01, the most obvious source of cholera global. The vaccine is administered in approximately 3 oz of fluid. It's about 80% effective in people challenged three months. The vaccine (one-dose or single-dose) ought to be administered at least 10 weeks prior to the patient traveling into a cholera-endemic location.

International Epidemics And Effect Of Cholera

International Epidemics

Threats can intensify epidemics in states and in refugee camps.

Outbreaks with higher prices are the outcome. For instance, in the wake of the Rwanda crisis in 1994, outbreaks of cholera caused at least 48 000 instances and 23 800 deaths in a month at the refugee camps in Goma, the Congo. Although rarely so fatal, outbreaks are still of significant public health issues, causing significant socioeconomic disturbance in addition to lack of life. In 2001, WHO and its associates in the Global Outbreak Alert and Response Network engaged in the affirmation of 41 cholera outbreaks in 28 nations. Throughout history, outbreaks of cholera have all around the world affected inhabitants. Records in Hippocrates (460-377 BC) and Galen (129-216 AD) already described a disease that may have been cholera, along with many hints implying a cholera-like malady was also called at the regions of the Ganges River since antiquity. Contemporary understanding about cholera, however, dates only from the start of the 19th century when scientists started to make progress towards a better comprehension of the causes of the disorder and its proper treatment. The 1st pandemic, or worldwide epidemic, began in 1817 from the endemic region in South-East Asia, then reached further areas of the world. Back in 1961, the 7th cholera pandemic tide started in Indonesia and propagated quickly to other countries in Asia, Europe, Africa, and in 1991 into Latin America, which was liberated of cholera for more than 1 century. The disease spread quickly in Latin America, causing almost 400 000 reported instances and more than 4 thousand deaths in 16 countries of the Americas that year. Back in 1992, a serogroup -- a derivative of this EI Tor biotype -- appeared from Bangladesh and caused an epidemic. Designated V. cholerae

41

0139 Bengal, the brand-new serogroup has been discovered in 11 nations and additionally warrants surveillance. The chance of a pandemic can't be excluded while no evidence can be obtained to estimate the importance of the improvements. EI Tor, by way of instance, then acquired virulence to induce the pandemic and was initially isolated as a virulent strain in 1905.

Economic And Societal Impact

Along with human suffering, cholera outbreaks may impede growth in the communities, disrupt the arrangement, and cause anxiety. Unjustified responses by other nations include restricting or curtailing traveling from nations or import restrictions on certain foods. The cholera epidemic in Peru in 1991 cost the nation $770 million US dollars because of food trade embargoes and consequences on tourism.

Chapter 2: Influenza, Spanish Flu (1918-1920)

Influenza, universally recognized as "the flu," is a disease brought on by RNA viruses (Orthomyxoviridae family) that contaminate the respiratory region of many animals, birds, and people. In most individuals, the disease leads to the individual getting a fever, nausea, headache, and malaise (tired, no energy). A few folks may also complain of a sore throat, vomiting, and nausea. Nearly all people have influenza symptoms for approximately 1-2 months before recovering. But, in comparison with many other viral respiratory infections, like the frequent cold, influenza (flu) disease can lead to a more serious illness with a mortality rate (death rate) of about 0. 1 percent of individuals infected with the virus. The aforementioned is the standard situation for the annual happening of the "traditional" or "seasonal" flu strains. These outbreaks occur since the virus is now altered in a substantial way: every time a part of the population is exposed to a flu strain where the population has little if any immunity. These outbreaks are often termed epidemics. Unusually severe global outbreaks (pandemics) have happened many times in the previous hundred years because the flu virus has been discovered in 1933. With an examination of tissue that is preserved, the worst flu pandemic (also termed as the Spanish influenza or Spanish flu) happened in 1918 when the virus generated between 40-100 million deaths globally, with a mortality rate estimated to vary from 2%-20%. Back in April 2009, a new flu strain with little if any resistance was isolated from people in Mexico. It quickly spread across the world so quickly that the WHO announced this influenza strain (first termed publication H1N1 influenza A swine flu, frequently later called to H1N1 or swine flu) because the origin of a pandemic on June 11, 2009. This was the earliest flu pandemic in 41 decades. Luckily, there was a global response that comprised vaccine manufacturing, fantastic hygiene practices (particularly hand washing), and also the virus (H1N1) caused much less morbidity and mortality than was anticipated and predicted. The WHO announced the pandemic's ending on Aug. 2010, 10, since it fit the standards of the WHO. Researchers identified a brand-new influenza-related viral strain, H3N2, in 2011, but this breed has generated just about 330 ailments with a single passing in the U. S. Since 2003, a different strain, H5N1, a bird flu virus, which caused 650 ailments, was discovered by researchers. This virus hasn't yet been discovered by the U. S. and readily spreads among individuals compared to other influenza strains. Regrettably, individuals infected with H5N1 have a higher death rate (roughly 60 percent of infected men and women die). H5N1 does not transfer from person to person like the influenza viruses. The latest statistics for your mortality (death rates) from flu rate (death rate) for the USA in 2016 suggests that mortality from influenza varies from year to year. Death rates estimated from the CDC vary throughout 2012-2013 during 2011-2012, estimating about 56,000. At the 2017-2018 seasons, deaths reached a high: approximately 79,000. Resulting in the increased or refused to relatives, experts recommended that a big proportion of individuals went unvaccinated, leading to the amount of deaths. This bacterium may lead to lung infections in children and babies, and it causes eye, ear, sinus, joint, along with some other ailments, but it doesn't cause the flu. Another term that is perplexing is stomach flu. This expression describes a Gastrointestinal tract disease but isn't a respiratory disease like flu (influenza). Influenza viruses don't cause the stomach flu (gastroenteritis). Another name difficulty is with the illness swine influenza. Swine influenza is an illness that infects the expression swine flu, although pigs were implemented to some flu strain, which also can infect people (H1N1). In the pig, the 2018-19 variant of this virus (not infecting people thus far) murdered the huge bulk of pigs In China, forcing that nation's pork. The strain has been discovered in South Korea. Although originally symptoms of flu may mimic those of a cold, it is more painful with symptoms of fever, fatigue, and respiratory congestion. Colds can be brought on by over 100 distinct virus types, but just flu viruses (and subtypes) A, B, and C cause the flu. Additionally, colds don't lead to life-threatening illnesses. Although, serious illnesses such as pneumonia infections with influenza viruses may contribute to death or pneumonia.

1889–1890 Flu Pandemic

The 1889-1890 influenza the "Asiatic flu" or "Russian flu," was a deadly flu pandemic which killed about 1 million individuals globally. It had been the century's last great outbreak. The most-reported impacts of the pandemic happened October 1889 --

December 1890, together with recurrences at March -- June 1891, November 1891 -- June 1892, winter 1893--1894 and ancient 1895. It isn't known for certain what agent was responsible for the pandemic. Since the 1950s it's been conjectured to become Influenza a virus subtype H2N2. A 1999 zero archaeological research claimed the breed to become Influenza A virus subtype H3N8. A 2005 genomic virological study theorized that the virus may have been not really a flu virus, but human coronavirus OC43.

Outbreak And Disperse

Contemporary transportation infrastructure helped the spread of this 1889 flu. The 19 biggest European countries, including the Russian Empire, had 202,887 kilometers of railroads and transatlantic travel by ship took less than seven (not substantially different than present travel time by air, given that the time scale of the worldwide spread of a pandemic). First reported in Bukhara, Russian Empire, in May 1889, by November that year the epidemic had reached Saint Petersburg. In four months it had spread throughout the Northern Hemisphere. Deaths appeared in Saint Petersburg about 1 December 1889, also in the USA during the week of 12 January 1890. The period between summit mortality and the earliest instance was five months. In Malta, the Asiatic Flu took connection between January 1889 and March 1890, with a fatality rate of 4 percent (39 deaths), along with a resurgence on January-May 1892 with 66 deaths (3. 3% case fatality). When this flu began, whether it was contagious was debated, but its quick action and pervasiveness across all climates and terrains proved that it was. A consequence of the influenza in Malta is that flu became, for the time, a modifiable disease.

Symptoms

The symptoms of flu are similar to that of those with the indications being that of pains and chills, cold, and flu can emerge a one to 3 times following infection.

Symptoms include:

- Fever (sudden onset) and chills
- Dry cough, sore throat, and hoarseness
- Muscular aches and pains, such as headache and earache
- Watering reddened eyes, face, and mouth
- Nausea (feeling sick) and lack of desire
- Runny and blocked nose, or sinus congestion (more prevalent in ordinary colds)
- Sometimes, diarrhea or stomach pains

The symptoms of flu are a combination of the indicators of a frequent cold (but more acute), together with that of those signs of pneumonia, fatigue, and muscle pain. Ordinarily, it is combined with a fever and cough – a fantastic sign of the flu. In healthy people, the body's immune system can last as many as two weeks and naturally fights the flu. It's predictable that among 30 to 50 percent of flu infections don't have any symptoms. A definite diagnosis can be made using the rapid molecular assay evaluation, which can rapidly diagnose flu by carrying a nasal swab over the initial four weeks of symptomatic beginning. All these assays check for viral antigens (of those viruses mentioned below) and may provide results within half an hour.

Symptoms of this disease included fatigue, followed by a reduction of desire, dry cough, gut troubles, then excessive perspiration. Then, the organs could become affectd, causing pneumonia to grow. Humphries clarifies that pneumonia, or other respiratory problems caused by influenza, are often the key causes for death. This explains why it is hard to determine specific numbers killed by the influenza, as the recorded cause of death was something aside from the flu. From the summer of 1918, the virus rapidly spread to other states in Europe. Vienna, Budapest, and Hungary were enduring, and parts of Germany and France likewise influenced. Many kids in Berlin schools were reported sick and absent from school, and absences in armament factories decreased manufacturing. From June 25, 1918, Britain had been reached by the influenza outbreak in Spain. Back in July, the outbreak was hitting on the London textile exchange challenging, with a single mill having 80 from 400 employees go home ill in 1 day alone, based on "The Spanish Influenza Pandemic of 1918-1919: New Perspectives" (Rutledge, 2003). Back in London, reports on government employees absent on account of the influenza range from 25 to 50 percent of their workforce. The outbreak had turned into a pandemic. On August 1918, six Canadian sailors died on the St. Lawrence River. At precisely the exact same month, instances reported among the Swedish military, then in the nation's civilian population and among South Africa's laboring population. From September, the flu had reached the U. S. during the Boston harbor.

Causes

These viruses are airborne and consequently distributed through the air by coughing, ejecting roughly half a million virus particles. Influenza A and B are responsible for seasonal flu, whereas hepatitis C just causes mild symptoms. Influenza A is in charge of more serious pandemics. Influenza A is mostly hosted in wild aquatic creatures that normally cause 'bird-flu' in domestic and wild bird populations, in addition to the occasional human flu pandemic. Influenza A virushas been categorized by subtype according to two surface proteins: hem agglutinin (H) and neuraminidase (N). The several kinds of N and H are numbered and there are 11 different NA subtypes and 18 H subtypes. It is the combination of those proteins that determines which subtype the influenza A virus belongs to, e. g. , H1N1 (Spanish Flu 1918 and 2009) or H5N1 (Bird Flu 2004). Influenza A can be incredibly diverse and has a higher mutation rate, hence the immunity in humans throughout life. Influenza B is exclusive to people. It's just 1 subtype and even though there's antigenic drift leading to various breeds of Influenza B. There's not any antigenic change, so individuals typically have a greater degree of resistance to it from youth. Influenza C includes one species which may affect pigs, dogs, and people. Influenza C causes infections in kids. Even though a fourth category of flu virus was discovered in 2011, it seems to be more limited to cows and pigs, although there's concern that it might develop into an emerging disease hazard to cattle workers later on. When an individual has become infected, based on the kind and harmful properties of this breed, the disease may occur along various areas of the lymph system, or from different cells. Usually, humans only have particular enzymes which can permit flu viruses to infiltrate cells inside the lungs and throat (cleavage of both hem agglutinin) and consequently can't infect other organs or tissues, but more seriously virulent strains like H5N1 may also bind to receptors considerably deeper inside the lungs, and consequently have the ability to cause more severe symptoms such as pneumonia, in comparison to those that bind to the upper respiratory tracts and have a tendency to be less intense.

Treatment, Prevention & Control

Individuals suffering from it need to isolate themselves and avoid close contact with other people in the attempt to restrict the spread of this virus. Basic preventative approaches like washing the hands with warm soap and water, the usage of cells when coughing, and blowing the nose and not stockpiling used cells might be a fantastic beginning in restricting spread. The ideal plan of action for somebody who has flu is to sleep, keep warm, drink lots of fluids, choose OTC (over the counter) drugs like paracetamol or aspirin to treat aches, pains and fever signs. OTC medication mixes may be obtained but should not be taken with paracetamol together since they include it. As flu is viral, antibiotics won't have any influence on the disease or change the results at all, unless there's a secondary bacterial disease after flu infection. The sole treatment of flu is antivirals, particularly within the first 48 hours of disease, but lots of virus strains are resistant to traditional antivirals. The principal antivirals used comprise oseltamivir (75mg twice daily for 5 days) or zanamivir (10mg as 2x 5mg puff inhalations, twice per day for 5 days). These antivirals may also be utilized as chemoprophylaxis brokers to stop or decrease the seriousness of flu if contaminated (in high-risk classes). Healthy people may fight the disease naturally but high-risk groups, such as pregnant women, kids and the elderly, might be awarded antivirals. Particular groups of individuals might qualify for the free influenza vaccine in the United Kingdom on a yearly basis in the run-up to sunlight. These include those within age 65, pregnant women, obese people, careers and house employees, kids of college-age, or people with chronic ailments. It's necessary to stress that the 'flu-jab' doesn't guarantee protection against seasonal flu. It lessens the danger of disease and/or complications of disease in risk groups. A new flu vaccine has to be made annually for every flu season according to the most frequent variations of the preceding year as a result of elevated mutation rates of these germs.

How Can Flu Spread?

How Do You Get Flu?

Flu spreads from person to person, either directly or indirectly. Influenza transmission occurs through droplets. Mass-produced by coughing, sneezing, or perhaps speaking, these droplets land close or at the mouth or the nose of uninfected men and women, and the illness could spread to them. The illness can spread directly to other people if contaminated droplets land on dishes, utensils, clothes, or any surface which uninfected individuals then touch. When the infected person touches their mouth or nose, by way of instance, they move or spread the illness to others or themselves.

The Secret To Influenza (Influenza) Avoidance

Flu Vaccine

Flu vaccination can prevent the majority of the disease. The CDC's present Advisory Committee on vaccination Practices (ACIP) issued recommendations for everybody 6 weeks old and older, which don't have any contraindications to vaccination, to get a flu vaccine every year. Flu vaccine (flu vaccine produced from inactivated and occasionally referred no infective virus or virus elements) is especially suggested for people that are at elevated risk for developing severe complications from influenza disease. Other hygiene approaches might reduce or prevent some people from getting the flu. For instance, preventing kissing, handshakes, and sharing drinks or food with contaminated individuals and preventing touching surfaces such as sinks and other things managed by people with influenza are great preventative measures. Rinsing one's hands with heated water and cleanser, or by using an alcohol-based hand sanitizer regularly can help prevent the disease. People with influenza should avoid coughing or coughing on uninfected individuals; rapid hugs are most likely okay so long as there isn't any contact with mucosal surfaces or droplets which could contain the virus.

How Effective Is The Flu Vaccine?

Vaccine efficacy changes from 1 individual to another. Long-term studies of strong young adults have found the flu vaccine to be 70%-90% effective in preventing disease. From the elderly and people with certain chronic medical conditions like HIV, the vaccine is most frequently less effective in preventing disease. Studies reveal that the vaccine reduces hospitalization by about 70% and death by about 85% among the elderly who aren't in nursing homes. Among nursing home residents, vaccine can decrease the probability of hospitalization by about 50%, the chance of pneumonia by about 60%, and the hazard of death by 75%-80%. This happens since the vaccine has to be made months before the influenza season starts, so the vaccine was created by projecting and deciding upon the most likely viral strains to include in the vaccine. If drift contributes to altering the circulating virus in the breeds used in the vaccine, efficiency may be reduced. The vaccine is possible to prevent death and complications and to lower the intensity of the disease, according to the CDC.

Why It Is That People Will Need To Get The Flu (Influenza) Vaccine Each Year?

Although a couple of virus strains that are distinct circulate at any particular time, individuals can continue to become sick with the flu. The cause of this susceptibility is that flu viruses are mutating, through the mechanics of drift and antigenic shift. Every year, researchers upgrade the vaccine to incorporate the latest influenza virus strains that are infecting people globally. The reason why influenza genes change is just one reason individuals need to get the vaccine. Another motive is that antibody created by the host in response to this vaccine decreases over time, and antibody levels are generally low annually, following vaccination so even when the exact same vaccine is used, it can work as a booster taken to elevate immunity. A lot of individuals still refuse to get flu shots due to misunderstandings, anxiety, "since I never get any shots," or even only a belief that should they get the flu, then they'll succeed. These are a few of the motives but there are more. The U. S., along with other nations' inhabitants, will need to be educated concerning genders; at least they ought to understand that protected vaccines have existed for years (measles, mumps, chickenpox, and just a vaccine for cholera), and as adults, they frequently must get a vaccine-like shot to check for tuberculosis exposure or to shield themselves from tetanus. The influenza vaccines are as secure since shots and these vaccines are accepted by the general public. Consequently, attempts will need to be made to create flu vaccines that are annual and acceptable as vaccines. Susceptible men and women will need to see that the vaccines manage them a substantial opportunity to reduce or stop this possibly debilitating disorder, hospitalization, and, in some cases, a deadly flu-caused disease.

Identification Of Virus Subtype Accountable

Researchers have attempted to identify the subtypes of Influenza accountable for the 1889--1890, 1898--1900 and 1918 epidemics. Originally, this function was mostly based on "seroarcheology"-- that the discovery of antibodies to influenza disease from the sera of older individuals --and it had been believed the 1889--1890 pandemic was caused by Influenza A subtype H2, the 1898--1900 outbreak by subtype H3, along with also the 1918 pandemic by subtype H1. Together with the affirmation of H1N1 since the origin of the 1918 influenza pandemic after identification of H1N1 compounds in exhumed corpses, reanalysis of all zero archeological data has signaled that Influenza A subtype H3 (maybe the H3N8 subtype) is a more probable cause for its 1889--1890 pandemic. Following the SARS outbreak, virologists began sequencing and comparing animal and human coronaviruses and contrast of 2 virus strains at the Beta coronavirus 1 species, Bovine coronavirus and Human coronavirus OC43 suggested they had a recent common ancestor from the late 19th century, with various methods yielding most likely dates around 1890. The authors theorized that an introduction of the strain into the inhabitants may have led to the outbreak.

An Ending, For Now

By February 1890, based on contemporary accounts, the flu had mostly disappeared from the U. S. Difficult as the pandemic had been, the country had gotten off lucky compared to Europe. New York City recorded the maximum number of deaths, even together with 2,503, though Boston, using a smaller population, was harder to hit a per-capita basis. The complete U. S. death toll was only under 13,000, according to the U. S. Census Office, from about 1 million globally. However, the Russian influenza wasn't entirely finished. It returned many times in subsequent years. Luckily, a large section of the U. S. population was resistant by then, subjected to it through its very first trip. These days, the flu is forgotten, overshadowed by a lot more devastating flu of 1918. But it did give Americans a preview of life—and death—in an increasingly interconnected world.

Spanish Flu (1918-1920)

The influenza, also called the 1918 influenza pandemic, an Influenza pandemic brought on by the H1N1 influenza a virus. Lasting during spring or early summer 1919 from spring 1918, 500 million people -- a third of the planet's population – was infected by it. The death toll estimated to have been anywhere from as large as 100 million, and 17 million to 50 million, which makes it among the deadliest pandemics in history. To keep sanity, World War I censor diminished historical reports of mortality and illness in Germany, the UK, France, and the USA. Newspapers were free to report that the epidemic's effects in neutral Spain, like the grave illness of King Alfonso XIII, and such stories generated a false belief of Spain as particularly hard hit. This gave rise to the title "Spanish" influenza. Ancient and epidemiological data are insufficient to find with certainty that the pandemics geographical source, with varying perspectives about its place. Most flu outbreaks kill the incredibly young and the incredibly old, using a greater survival rate for all those in between, but the Spanish influenza pandemic led to a greater than expected mortality rate for adults. Researchers supply several explanations for its high mortality rate of the 1918 flu pandemic. Some investigations have proved that the virus is especially deadly because it activates a cytokine storm, which ravages the more powerful immune system of young adults. In contrast, a 2007 evaluation of health care journals in the length of the pandemic discovered that the viral disease was no more competitive than earlier flu strains. Rather, malnourishment, overcrowded medical camps and hospitals, and inadequate hygiene all affected by the current war, encouraged bacterial super infection. This super infection killed all the victims, normally. The 1918 "Spanish" influenza was the first of 2 pandemics brought on by the H1N1 influenza A virus. The next was the 2009 swine flu pandemic.

What Triggered The Spanish Flu?

The outbreak started in 1918 War I, and historians today think that the battle might have been partially responsible for distributing the virus. In the Western Front, soldiers living in moist, dirty, and crowded conditions became sick. This is a consequence of immune systems from malnourishment. Their disorders, which are called "agrip," were contagious, and dispersed among the positions. Within around three times of getting sick, many soldiers will begin to feel better, but not all could make it. Throughout the summer of 1918, as soldiers started to return home on leave, they brought with them the unnoticed virus that made them sick. The virus spread throughout villages, towns, and cities at the soldiers' home states. A lot of those infected civilians and soldiers did not recover. The virus was toughest on young adults between the ages of 20 and 30 who had previously been healthy. In 2014, a new concept about the roots of this virus showed it appeared in China according to National Geographic. Previously undiscovered records connected the influenza into the transport of Chinese laborers, the Chinese Labour Corps, across Canada in 1917 and 1918. The laborers were mostly plantation workers from distant parts of rural China, based on Mark Humphries' book "The Last Plague" (University of Toronto Press, 2013). They spent six days in sealed train containers since they hauled throughout the nation before continuing into France. In all, over 90,000 employees mobilized into the front.

Humphries clarifies that in 1 count of 25,000 Chinese laborers in 1918, a few 3,000 stopped their Canadian travel in medical care. Now, due to racial stereotypes, their ailment blamed "Chinese laziness" and Canadian physicians did not take the employees' symptoms severely. From the time that the laborers came in northern France in early 1918, many were ill, and countless were shortly perishing.

Why Was It Known As The Spanish Flu?

Spain was among the countries where the outbreak was recognized, but historians think that this was due to wartime censorship. Spain was a neutral state during the war and did not impose rigorous censorship of its own media, which may so freely publish ancient reports of this disease. Because of this, people kindly believed that the disease was unique to Spain, and the title "Spanish influenza" stuck. In late September 1918, a Spanish news agency sent word to Reuters' London office notifying the news agency that "a peculiar type of illness of epidemic character has emerged in Madrid. The outbreak is of a gentle character, zero deaths reported," according to Henry Davies' book "The Spanish Flu," (Henry Holt & Co. , 2000). Within a couple of weeks of this report, more than 100,000 people had become infected with the flu. The illness struck the king of Spain, Alfonso XIII, together with major politicians. Between 30 and 40 percent of individuals who lived or worked in restricted areas, like schools, barracks, and government buildings, became contaminated. Service on the Madrid tram system needed to decrease, and the telegraph service was upset, in both instances because there were not enough health workers available to do the job. Services and supplies could not keep up with demand. The word "Spanish flu" quickly took hold in Britain. Based on Niall Johnson's book "Britain and the 1918-19 Influenza Pandemic" (Rout ledge, 2006), the British media blamed the influenza outbreak in Spain in the Spanish sport: ". . . the arid, windy Spanish spring is an unpleasant and unhealthy period," read a single post at The Times. It had showed that the winds in Spain were spreading dust, meaning Britain climate could block the flu.

How Many People Died?

From the start of 1919, Influenza was diminishing. Nations left devastated in the aftermath of the epidemic, as medical professionals were not able to stop the spread of this illness. The pandemic echoed what had occurred 500 years before, when the Black Death wreaked havoc across the world. Nancy Bristow's publication "American Pandemic: The Lost Worlds of the 1918 Influenza Epidemic" (Oxford University Press, 2016) clarifies the virus influenced as many as 500 million people across the planet. Now, this stood for a third of the population. As many as 50 million people died from the virus, even though the real figure is much greater. Bristow estimates the virus-infected up to 25 percent of the U. S. inhabitants, and among members of the U. S. Navy, this amount reached around 40 percent, possibly because of conditions of functioning at sea. The flu had killed 200,000 Americans from the end of October 1918. Bristow also asserts the pandemic murdered 675,000 Americans. The influence on the populace was so acute, the American life expectancy decreased by 12 decades. Statistics piled up to such an extent that cemeteries overrun, and households needed to dig graves to their relatives. The deaths made a lack of farmworkers, which influenced. As in Britain, a lack of resources and staff set solutions, such as waste collection. The earthquake spread into South America, Africa, Asia, and the South Pacific. In India, the mortality rate reached 50 deaths per 1,000 individuals -- a figure that was shocking.

The International Death Count Of This Influenza Now

To have a circumstance for the severity of flu pandemics, it might be extremely helpful to be aware of the departure count of a normal flu season. Recent estimates for the yearly number of deaths from the flu are 400,000 deaths each year. Paget et al (2019) show a mean of 389,000 having an uncertainty range of 294,000 from 518,000. This implies that in the past few decades the flu has been responsible for the passing of 0.0052 percent of the world population -- just one individual for every 18,750. 5 Even compared to the minimal quote, because of the death count of the Spanish influenza (17. 4 million), more than a century past that led to a death rate 182 -times greater than the current baseline.

Asian Flu Pandemic 1957--1958

1957 influenza pandemic, also Asian flu of 1957, an epidemic of flu that was found in East Asia and spread to nations. The 1957 influenza outbreak caused an estimated 1 million to 2 million deaths and is regarded to have been the most acute of the three flu pandemics of the 20th century. A virus caused the 1957 epidemic. Studies have suggested that this virus was a reasserting (mixed species) strain, originating from strains of avian flu and human flu viruses. From the 1960s the H2N2 strain bought a series of genetic alterations, a process. Epidemics generated by these modifications. Following 10 decades of development, the 1957 flu virus vanished, replaced through antigenic change by a new influenza a subtype, H3N2 that gave rise to the 1968 influenza pandemic. In the very first weeks of the 1957 influenza pandemic, the virus spread across China and surrounding areas. From midsummer the United States, in which it has infected men and women had reached by it. However, a lot of cases of the disease reported in elderly girls and children. This upsurge in cases has been the consequence of a second wave of disease that struck on the Northern Hemisphere. At that point, the pandemic was widespread in the UK. December had a total of several 3,550 deaths reported in Wales and England. The next wave was devastating, and in the USA a death had happened from March 1958. Comparable to the 1968 Pandemic, the 1957 epidemic was correlated with variation. Others underwent complications like pneumonia while some people have undergone only minor symptoms, such as cough and mild fever. The growth of a vaccine from the virus along with also the availability of antibiotics to treat infections restricted mortality and the spread of this pandemic.

History

The strain of the virus that caused the pandemic A Virus subtype H2N2 was a recombination of avian influenza (from geese) and human flu viruses. There was resistance in the populace since it turned out to be a novel strain of this virus. The first cases reported in Guizhou in late 1956 or even February 1957, and have reported at the neighboring state of Yunnan prior to the end of February. On 17 April, The Times reported that "a flu outbreak has influenced tens of thousands of Hong Kong residents." From the end of the month, Singapore experienced an outbreak of this influenza, which appeared with deaths in mid-May. Back in Taiwan, mid-May influenced 100,000 and a million cases were endured by India. In June, the pandemic reached the United Kingdom. From June 1957 it reached the USA, where diseases were caused by it. A number of those changed were United States Navy employees at destroyers docked at Newport Naval Station, in addition to military recruits everywhere. The very first tide peaked in October (among kids who returned to college) and the next wave, in January and February 1958, among older men and women, which had been more deadly. Microbiologist Maurice Hilleman alerted by photos of these affected by the virus in Hong Kong. He bought samples of this virus. The Public Health Service introduced the virus civilizations to vaccine producers on 12 May 1957, along with a vaccine entered trials at Fort Ord on 26 July and Lowry Air Force Base on 29 July. The number of deaths peaked the week ending 17 October, with 600 reported in Wales and England. The vaccine was first available in precisely the exact same month in the UK. Its installation helped have the pandemic, even though it was available only in limited amounts. H2N2 flu virus continued to circulate until 1968, as it changed via influenza virus subtype H3N2.

Mortality Estimates

The case fatality rate of Asian influenza was 0.67 percent. The disorder had estimated to have a 3 percent rate of complications and 0.3 percent mortality in the United Kingdom. It may lead to pneumonia alone, without the existence of secondary bacterial disease. It might have infected as many more individuals, however, the vaccine improved health care, as well as the creation of antibiotics led to a lower mortality rate. The CDC quotes 1. 1 million deaths globally. According to a study in the Journal of Infectious Diseases, the excess mortality occurred in Latin America. 70,000 to 116,000 people died in the USA. In 1958, it had estimated that 14,000 people had died of influenza in the United Kingdom. It caused ailments contributing to college closures and dispersing in schools but has been fatal. The virus was deadly in the elderly, women, and those with preexisting heart and lung disease. Based on a study from Barbara Sands, several of the mortality attributed to the great leap forward might have brought on by the 1957 flu.

Chapter 3: Typhus (1618-2018)

Typhus is a disorder brought on by germs (mainly Rickettsia typhi or R. prowazekii). There are two big kinds of typhus: endemic (or murine typhus) and epidemic typhus -- bacterial diseases trigger both. The germs are tough to cultivate and small. They were believed to be viruses. The disorder occurs after germs (Rickettsia) move to people, typically by vectors like lice or fleas, which have obtained the bacteria from animals like cats, rats, opossums, raccoons, and other creatures. Endemic typhus (mostly due to R. typhi) can also be termed murine typhus and "prison fever." "Endemic typhus" also suggests an area has animal inhabitants (usually rats, rodents (or rabbits), which have members of its inhabitants always infected with R. typhi that via flea vectors can independently infect people. Epidemic typhus (due to R. prowazekii) is the more severe type of typhus. Additionally, it has been termed irregular or recrudescent typhus. "Epidemic typhus" also suggests a few critters, (usually rats) through lice vectors, may independently infect large numbers of people quickly when specific environmental conditions exist (poor hygiene, crowded human living conditions) together with the more sterile R. prowazekii. Epidemic typhus includes a milder type termed Brill-Zinsser disorder, which happens if R. prowazekii bacteria reactivate at an individual formerly infected with epidemic typhus. There's a confusion surrounding the word "typhus. " A lot of individuals equate typhus with typhoid (typhoid fever), which can be erroneous. There's confusion for numerous factors. Both disorders have in common the symptom of hypertension, and also the significant species of Rickettsia, which triggers endemic typhus remains termed "typhi. "The causes, transmission, pathology, and treatment of those diseases are different. Fever is caused by salmonella species, which is irrelevant to Rickettsia. Perplexing is that the expression scrub typhus, which describes a distinct although, related disease brought on by the parasite Orientiatsutsugamushi that is mobile. This disorder is connected to typhus and endemic to South America and some parts of Africa, however results from another genus and species of bacteria and can be transmitted with another vector (fleas). This article's intention is to inform the reader about both global variants of typhus, endemic along with also the more acute epidemic typhus.

The History Of Typhus

Among the earliest descriptions of this disease (likely of epidemic typhus) describing rash, sores, delirium, and roughly 17,000 deaths of Spanish troops had been through the siege of Granada at 1489. Descriptions above period termed jail strain or the illness goal. In 1759 authorities estimated roughly 25 percent of all prisoners in England expired of fever each year. From the smoke or stupor due to the symptom of delirium which could grow, the disorder was termed typhus in 1760. Typhus epidemics have been linked to inadequate living conditions and raged throughout Europe. By way of instance, some historians estimate more of Napoleon's troops were murdered by typhus than by soldiers during their retreat from

Moscow in 1812. The Americas and Ireland recorded epidemics. From outbreaks, over 100,000 Irish expired from the 1830s. In the U. S. between 1837 to 1873, epidemics were documented in Philadelphia, Concord, Baltimore, and Washington, D. C. Henrique, a Brazilian physician, found that the reason for epidemic typhus in 1916 while performing research on typhus at Germany. But still, more than 3 million deaths were attributed to typhus during and following World War I. Delousing channels were often set up to attempt to decrease the speed of typhus disease and death among soldiers and civilians. Though a typhus vaccine has been designed prior to World War II, typhus epidemics continued, particularly in German absorption camps throughout the Holocaust (Anne Frank died in a camp at age 15 from typhus). Finally, DDT was used to kill lice in the conclusion of World War II, and also just a couple of epidemics (Africa, Middle East, Eastern Europe, and Asia) have happened since then. Due to toxicity, DDT was banned from the U. S. since 1972. Endemic typhus appears to be rising or possibly has been recognized and properly diagnosed more frequently from the U. S. A good example would be the following: Though endemic typhus is generally found in cooler surroundings, in 2011, Travis County, Texas, (such as Austin, Texas) was announced to be widespread for murine (endemic) typhus with 53 cases diagnosed. California has typhus. With the disorder -- the first time, Galveston County, Texas, reported 17 people in 2018. Police suggest a lot more people might be infected but have never been diagnosed.

What Causes Typhus? Can Typhus Spread?

The root of typhus is Coccobacilli-shaped germs, members of the genus Rickettsia which are intracellular parasites of several creatures and use the elements within the cell to multiply and survive. Typhus is occasionally tagged as tick-borne typhus or typhus. They are hard to cultivate since they generally grow inside cells that they infect. Sometimes, the bacteria may become dormant in cells that are infected, and years after, again start to multiply (inducing Brill-Zinsser disorder). Normally, typhus follows an animal (rat, mouse) into vector (louse, flea) cycle. If the vectors come in close proximity to 14, Individuals are infected usually. Both Rickettsia species in charge of both chief kinds of typhus are Rickettsia prowazekii, the reason for epidemic typhus, and R. typhi, the reason for endemic typhus. But, R. felis, yet another species usually seen in kitty and cat fleas (Ctenocephalidesfelis), has been associated with individuals with endemic typhus also. Epidemic typhus normally spreads to individuals in body lice feces infected with R. prowazekii or sometimes from animal droppings infected with these bacteria. Endemic typhus normally spreads to humans by flea stool or animal droppings containing R. typhi or even R. felis. The flea or louse (Pediculushumanus) sting causes itching and scratching and can permit the bacteria to enter the bite or scratch place in the epidermis. Indirect person-to-person transmission of rickettsia can happen if infected fleas or lice infect one individual who develops the illness and subsequently the infected pests or pests proceed from person to person by direct contact or through shared clothing. Generally, head lice which differ in body lice, don't transmit Rickettsia.

Which Are Typhus Risk Factors?

Risk factors include living in or visiting regions where the illness is endemic. These include many port towns in which rat populations are large, and regions where garbage accumulates and hygiene might be reduced. Disaster zones, displaced camps, poverty-stricken places, and other related scenarios that allow rodents to develop intimate contact with individuals represent the best threats. These are the exact same sort of conditions that result in outbreaks of cholera, tuberculosis, and viral diseases like flu. Spring and summer months are full of fleas and ticks, but diseases can happen at any time of the year.

Which Are Typhus Signs And Symptoms?

Indicators of typhus grow within approximately 1 to 2 months after initial infection and might include a high fever (roughly 105 F), headache, malaise, nausea, vomiting, and nausea. A rash on the stomach and the torso begins approximately four to seven days following the symptoms above grow, as well as the rash spreads. Some individuals may also have a cough along with stomach pain, joint pain, and back pain. Symptoms can last for approximately two months and, barring death or complications (less than 2 percent perish), symptoms persist. Epidemic typhus symptoms, though similar to typhus, are becoming more intense. The rash may cover the whole body except the bottoms of their toes and the palms of their hands. Patients can develop further indicators of bleeding into the skin (petechiae), delirium, stupor, hypotension, and shock, which is life-threatening.

The Remedy For Typhus

Physicians recommend antibiotic treatment for both Epidemic typhus illnesses because early treatment with antibiotics (by way of instance, azithromycin, doxycycline, tetracycline, or chloramphenicol) can heal many people infected with bacteria. Consultation with a specialist is advised if typhus or epidemic typhus in women that were elderly is diagnosed. Delays in treatment may allow lung or nervous system problems to grow. Some patients may perish.

Is It Feasible To Stop Typhus? Can There Be A Typhus Vaccine?

Efforts to reduce typhus have been powerful when individuals can prevent contact with all the vectors that spread typhus (mostly lice and fleas) or fecal droppings from rodents. In locations where endemic typhus is present, or in outbreaks of epidemic typhus, attempts to take care of domestic animals to rid them of insects are great preventative measures. Many experts suggest that good sanitation, flea-control steps, and diminishing populations of mice, rats, and other creatures that can carry the germs and their vectors are successful. Use insect repellents and insecticides (for instance, 1 percent malathion or 1 percent permethrin) if lice and fleas live in the neighborhood atmosphere. In case the challenge is salty and lice clothing isn't feasible, the lice will be allowed by preventing any contact. There is no vaccine for epidemic or endemic typhus. The CDC doesn't recommend taking any antibiotics to prevent the disease.

Typhus Vs. Typhoid

Although they appear like typhoid and typhus are various ailments. Typhoid is a fungal disease. Folks get typhoid with a kind of salmonella bacteria that are found in food and water. Folks can contract typhoid in the stool of animals and people carrying the illness. Typhoid is infrequent in high-income countries, like the United States, although common in developing countries with inadequate sanitation.

These elements can help lessen the chance of typhoid disease:

- Frequent hand washing
- Appropriate food sanitation
- Using just sterile, purified water

Chapter 4: Smallpox(1614-2011)

Smallpox is an infectious disease of yesteryear that health care professionals removed by legislation. The illness, which spreads from person to person, is caused by the variola virus. Individuals became ill with a fever and a rash. As much as one-third of individuals with smallpox died. Samples of this virus exist in labs in Russia and the USA despite the disease being wiped out. This has caused concerns about the usage of this virus from biological warfare. Because of this, health care providers vaccinate some army personnel from smallpox.

The History Of Smallpox

Smallpox existed for more than 12,000 decades. Mummies from early Egypt revealed signs of disease, including the mummy of Ramses V. Smallpox entered the New World from the 16th century. Populations were decimated by smallpox since the inhabitants had no resistance to this disease. There are reports where American inhabitants were infected by people from the 18th century with blankets -- among the cases of biological warfare. There were 300M to 500M deaths compared to 100 million in tuberculosis. It wasn't until the end of the century when an effective technique of vaccination was designed. An English scientist named Edward Jenner found it. Jenner observed that milkmaids got an illness called cowpox, which appeared to make them resistant to smallpox. His vaccination plan involved moving the blister fluid from an individual with cowpox to some man who hadn't had smallpox (an obsolete procedure termed variolation). This gave the vulnerable individual a cowpox disease (that was generally mild) and hauled protection against smallpox. After a moment, there was very similar to cowpox a virus substituted at the vaccine. The last case of smallpox was in Somalia in 1977. Back in 1980, the World Health Organization (WHO) and the World Health Assembly certified the world was free from smallpox. Smallpox has been the first disorder to be eradicated. Efforts are underway to attempt to eliminate diseases like measles and polio. The WHO, post-eradication of this virus clinically (no more smallpox cases in the world), has supported all member countries to destroy any residual lab cultures of the virus. The growth of biological warfare technologies led to concerns whether individuals could weaponize smallpox to use in bioterrorism. The U. S. (CDC, Atlanta, Georgia) and Russia (Koltsovo) chose to keep their stockpiles if they were required to make novel offenses from a biological agent. Controversy has stirred up. The whole genome was sequenced, resulting in concerns that the virus could possibly be recreated when stocks have been ruined. Smallpox is a life-threatening illness (30 percent or greater death rate with acute hemorrhagic disease) and is among the list of future biological weapons believed to pose the best danger to public health. Brokers with this list include anthrax, plague, smallpox, botulism, tularemia, and viral hemorrhagic fevers.

What Causes Smallpox?

A poxvirus known as variola (Poxviridae family of germs, genus Orthopoxvirus) causes smallpox. Variola is a large virus that has DNA. The virus resides in massive amounts in several organs (kidneys, skin, spleen, liver, and other organs) of infected men and women. Death happens because of toxemia, considered to be caused by immune complexes hoping to respond to the number of particles. Variola disease occurs. There are two breeds known as variola major and variola minor (also called alastrim). According to the titles, variola major is more likely to cause severe illness and death compared to variola.

Risk Factors For Smallpox

Before, the significant risk factor for getting smallpox disease was close affiliation with another individual with smallpox who expelled droplets in sneezes and coughs. It was rare that patients might have contracted the illness from touching things that were contaminated and then moving viruses. Presently, the risk factors are currently operating in specialized labs that may have smallpox viruses in storage or become infected while either working together with the viruses (for instance, a poxvirus laboratory technician, vaccinator, or transporter) or employing the viruses as a biological weapon.

Incubation Period For Smallpox

The incubation period for smallpox is a bit more than a number of different viruses; symptoms grow approximately seven to 17 days following exposure.

How Does Smallpox Spread?

The transmission of smallpox is from person to person. Infectious droplets of saliva inhaled by someone else and then are expelled during coughing or sneezing. This normally necessitates close face-to-face contact and also is like the manner that mumps, measles, and influenza are dispersed. Normally, one person would infect roughly 60 percent of the household contacts. Infected items, for example, used silverware or heavily contaminated bedding, can carry adequate quantities of organisms to infect another individual if improperly managed, but this path of transmission is not as common.

The Signs And Smallpox Symptoms

Fever can be very significant and is the most frequent symptom. The fever is accompanied by indications like headache, chills, and body aches. Many times, the individual is too sterile to get out of bed (malaise). Within 24-48 hours, a rash starts to appear within the human body but particularly on the face, mouth, arms, and the thighs. Pharyngitis (painful throat), abdominal hurting, back throbbing, and sometimes vomiting may also grow. The eyes can be affected, resulting in possible blindness between survivors. Symptoms in children are alike to those in adults. The rash extends through phases as the disorder progresses and appears on the palms and soles. The rash consists, which becomes increased. The skin lesions quickly fill with fluid and might turn yellow, including pus (pus-filled lesions). Paradoxically, the rash might begin to fill with blood (hemorrhagic smallpox), and it can be a bad prognostic sign. The lesions drop off, leaving scars and finally scab over. One of the characteristics of smallpox is that the lesions in the body are at precisely the exact same stage of growth. Approximately one-third of individuals with smallpox died from the disease. Individuals who had even a mild rash or just a couple of lesions had a chance of dying. Diseases caused by the variola minor strain had been severe and death happened in only roughly 1 percent of cases. When smallpox was ordinary, a seasoned clinician could produce the identification by simply taking a look at the rash and analyzing the patient. Any instance that happens will be due to bioterrorism or biological warfare. In that event, delays or misdiagnoses could get the disease. Therefore, it's still essential for clinicians to have the ability to diagnose smallpox.

The Cure For Smallpox

Treatment for smallpox is reassuring, meaning that patients ought to keep hydrated, fever ought to be treated with acetaminophen (Tylenol) or a similar medicine, and the patient must be carefully tracked to establish whether there's a demand for blood pressure support. Even though there are no drugs shown to work against human disease, some drugs have shown promise in the lab, such as a derivative of the antiviral drug cidofovir (Vistide), its analogs, and the virus inhibitor ST-246. Rigorous airborne and contact isolation procedures should be followed closely if the individual is hospitalized; the area ought to have HEPA air filters and negative air pressure.

Might It Be Feasible To Reduce Smallpox?

Smallpox is a disease that is vaccine-preventable. Health researchers utilize a virus called vaccinia to generate the vaccine. The similarity between both of these titles (vaccine and vaccinia) isn't coincidental because smallpox has been the first disease to be prevented by vaccination. In 2007, a second-generation smallpox vaccine (ACAM2000) has been accredited. The vaccine includes live vaccinia virus but doesn't comprise any smallpox virus. It's not a shot and physicians administer it in a special way: a sharp, pronged piece of metal is dipped from the embryo and then utilized to prick the skin of the receiver. Doctors repeat this procedure many times. When effective, the site of vaccination will create tiny blisters which scab and heal, leaving a scar, consequently generating minor negative reactions (a procedure called scarification). Even though the blisters are busy, folks should keep the site clean and covered to avoid the vaccinia virus from spreading to other people. Many adults have a vaccine scar in their arms. Smallpox vaccine, such as other vaccines like the yellow fever vaccine, educates the immune system of the body to recall creating antibodies. There can be a degree of security, even decades following vaccination. However, revaccination is recommended by doctors. Vaccination after exposure provides some protection from disease. Health officials advocate vaccination since the disease was eradicated. Presently, laboratory workers who manage the smallpox virus and only chosen personnel get the vaccine. Adverse reactions are rare but are occasionally serious and possibly deadly. Complications occur in roughly 75 million adults. Because the vaccine includes live vaccinia virus, the virus can spread and infect the heart, causing myocarditis (disease of the heart muscle) or pericarditis (infection of the sac around the heart). The vaccine may also infect the brain (encephalitis) or attention or lead to a generalized rash. Complications result in about 1 individual for each million individuals, sometimes resulting in death. Complications are less prevalent in revaccination. People with skin circumstances, such as eczema and individuals with weak immune systems, are at greater risk for complications. Women shouldn't be vaccinated due to the possibility of death. Health researchers haven't analyzed the antiviral medication tecovirimat (Tpoxx) in people, but it had been quite powerful in animals in shielding them against monkey pox and rabbit pox, ailments that are linked to smallpox. No side effects were caused by the medication when safety-tested in 359 individuals. The development of this medication was done to be able to get treatment available in the event of a biological laboratory accident or to shield from a bioterror attack.

Chapter 5: Measles (1855-2005)

Measles is a tremendously transmittable, infectious disease instigated by the measles virus. Symptoms develop 10-12 days after exposure to an infected individual. The first symptoms typically include fever, frequently higher than 40 °C (104 °F), cough, runny nose, and inflamed eyes. White spots can form three or two days following the beginning of symptoms. A flat rash that begins on the face and spreads into the rest of the body begins after the beginning of symptoms. Frequent complications include nausea (in 8 percent of cases), middle ear disease (7%), and pneumonia (6%). These happen in part as a result of measles-induced immunosuppressant. Blindness, frequent seizures, or inflammation of the brain might happen. Other titles contain measles, rubeola, red measles, and morbilli. The two rubella, also called "German measles," and roseola are unique ailments brought on by unrelated viruses. Measles is an airborne disease that spreads through the coughs and sneezes of infected men and women. It could also increase across connection with nasal or mouth secretions. It is extremely contagious; nine out of ten people who are not immune and share living space with an infected person will be infected. Individuals are infectious prior to four days. The majority of individuals don't get the disease more than once. Testing for the virus in cases is essential for general health efforts. The measles vaccine is secure, capable of preventing the disease, and is delivered in conjunction. Vaccination resulted in an 80% reduction in deaths from measles between 2000 and 2017. Roughly 85% of kids globally having obtained their first dose as of 2017. When an individual has become infected, no particular treatment is available even though supportive care can improve results. Such care could consist of an oral rehydration solution (somewhat salty and sweet fluids), healthy food, and drugs to control the strain. Antibiotics must be prescribed in case bacterial infections, like ear infections or pneumonia. Vitamin A supplementation is recommended for kids. Roughly 20 million people per year are affected by measles from the regions of Asia and Africa. It may affect individuals of any era while considered a childhood disorder. Back in 1980, 2.6 million people died of it, and in 1990, 545,000 expired. From 2014, worldwide vaccination programs had decreased the amount of deaths from measles to 73,000. Rates of deaths and illnesses rose because of a reduction in immunization by 2017 to 2019. The danger of death among those infected is about 0.2 percent, but it may be around 10 percent in people with malnutrition. The majority are less than five years old. Measles isn't known to occur in animals.

Symptoms

The Indicators of Measles always consist of fever and at least of one of the 3 Cs:

- Infection
- Coryza, or runny nose
- Conjunctivitis

- Symptoms may appear about 9 to 11 days after initial infection.

Symptoms can include:

- Runny nose
- Dry hacking cough
- Conjunctivitis, or swollen eyelids and inflamed eyes
- Watery eyes
- Photophobia, or sensitivity to light
- Infection
- A malodorous reckless
- Koplik's spots, or very slight grayish-white marks, with bluish-white centers: in the mouth, interiors of cheeks, and throat
- indiscriminated body aches

There is repeatedly a temperature. This can range from acute, up to 40.6 degrees Centigrade. It may last several days, as soon as the rash appears, and it can fall and rise again. The rash looks approximately 3 to 4 times after symptoms. This will last for more than a week. The rash usually begins behind the ears and spreads across the neck and the head. After a few days, it spreads to the respite of the body, containing the legs. As the spots grow, they frequently link together.

Most youth rashes aren't measles, but a child should visit a physician if:

- A parent supposes that the child may have measles
- Symptoms don't improve, or else they get worse
- The fever rise to over 38° Centigrade (°C) or 100. 4° Fahrenheit (°F)
- Other symptoms resolve, but the fever persists

Infection

Implications out of measles are common. Some could be serious. Individuals most at risk are the patients with a poor immune system, like those who have HIV, AIDS, leukemia, or a vitamin deficiency, young kids, and adults over 20 years of age. Individuals are more likely to have complications than healthy children.

Complications are:

- Infection
- vomiting
- Eye disease
- Respiratory tract ailments, for example, laryngitis and bronchitis
- Difficulty breathing
- Ear infections, which may result in permanent hearing loss
- Febrile seizures

Patients are more vulnerable to pneumonia. This may be deadly if not treated.

The next less typical complications are also possible:

- **Hepatitis:** Liver complications may occur in adults and in children that are taking any drugs.
- **Encephalitis:** This affects approximately 1 in every 1,000 patients with measles. It's an inflammation of the brain. It may happen rapidly later than measles, or several years later.
- **Thrombocytopenia,** or low platelet count, which affects the blood's ability to clot. The individual can bruise.
- **Squint**: Eye nerves and eye muscles can be influenced.

Unique And Possible Complications include:

- Neuritis, an illness of the optic nerve which may lead to vision loss
- Heart complications
- **Sub-acutesclerosingpan encephalitis (SSPE):** A brain disorder that could affect 2 out of every 100,000 individuals, years or months after measles infection. Death, motor abnormalities, cognitive problems, and convulsions might occur.
- Other nervous system complications consist of toxic encephalopathy, retro bulbar neuritis, transverse myelitis, and ascending myelitis.

Types

There are two types of measles:

- **Measles:** This is actually the conventional kind caused by the rubeola virus.
- **Rubella or German measles:** This is brought on by the rubella virus.

Rubella ordinarily exhibits as unimportant but presents more if a woman is pregnant. It's neither contagious nor as intense as ordinary measles. The measles, mumps, and rubella (MMR) vaccine include immunizations for both kinds.

Causes

Measles is caused by infection with the rubella virus. The virus resides in the mucus of the nose and throat of an infected adult or child. The disorder is infectious for 4 days before the rash appears, and it is still infectious for approximately 4 to 5 days after.

Infection spreads via:

- Physical contact with an infected individual
- Being close infected individuals if they sneeze or cough
- Touching a surface which has infected droplets of mucus, then placing fingers into the mouth, or rubbing the eyes or nose

The virus vestiges full of life on an object or surface for two hours.

How Does A Measles Infection Develop?

Whenever the virus enters the body, it multiplies in the back of the throat, lungs, and lymphatic system. It infects and reproduces in blood vessels, uterus, the urinary tract, and the nervous system. Symptoms arise between 9 and 11 days after infection, although the virus requires establishing itself. Anybody who has been vaccinated or infected is very likely to become sick if they breathe tainted droplets or are in close corporeal contact with an infected individual. Roughly 90 percent of individuals that aren't immune will create measles if they share a home with an infected individual.

Medication

There's not any particular kind of medication. If there are no difficulties, the doctor will suggest rest and plenteously of fluids to prevent dehydration. Indications ordinarily go away within 7 to 10 days.

The subsequent procedures can support:

- If the child's fever is high, they should be reserved cold, but not too cold. Tylenol or aspirin will help to control fever, aches, and pains. Aspirin should not be taken by kids under 16 years. A physician will advise concerning acetaminophen dose, as too much can harm the kid, particularly the liver. There's a great choice on the internet if you would like to buy Tylenol or ibuprofen.

- Individuals should preclude smoking nearby to the kid.

- Sunglasses, keeping the lights dim or the space dimmed may improve comfort levels, as measles raises sensitivity.

- Gently wash with a moist cloth when there's crustiness around the eyes.

- If cough will not alleviate, putting a humidifiers bowl of water from the area might help. If the child is more than 12 weeks, a glass of water with 2 teaspoons of honey plus a teaspoon of lemon juice can help. Don't give honey to babies.

- A fever may lead to dehydration, so the child should drink lots of fluids.

- A kid who's in the infectious stage ought to steer clear of college and avoid close contact with other people, particularly people who aren't immunized or haven't had measles.

- People that have kids less than 2 years who have measles and a vitamin A deficiency may benefit from vitamin supplements. These may help to prevent complications; however they should be obtained with the agreement of a doctor. If you would like to buy vitamin supplements, then there's a superb choice on the internet with thousands of consumer reviews.

Antibiotics won't help counter measles virus, but they may

sometimes be recommended if a further bacterial infectivity develops.

Identification

A doctor can typically diagnose measles by considering the indications and symptoms. A blood test will confirm the existence of the rubeola virus. Measles is a notifiable disease. The physician must notify the police of any suspected instances. If the patient is a child, then the health care provider will notify the school. A child with measles shouldn't return to school after the rash appears.

Prevention

People who already have measles are usually resistant and they are unlikely to get it again. People who are not resistant should consider the measles vaccine.

Measles Vaccination

In America, the measles, mumps, and rubella (MMR) vaccine is given at 12 to 15 weeks old, followed by a booster shot prior to entering school. When their mom's are resistant, newborns take their mother's immunity to get a month or two after birth, but the vaccine is recommended prior to age 12 months, as early as 6 weeks. This may take place if they are, or will likely be, in a region where there's a severe epidemic. The WHO estimates that measles vaccination plans resulted in a 79% drop in measles deaths worldwide from 2000 to 2015, preventing approximately 20.3 million deaths.

Adults don't need A vaccine at the U. S. if they:

- Were born or lived at the U. S. prior to 1957. From the U. S., unless they operate in a healthcare setting and don't have any evidence of resistance
- Received two MMR shots once they were 12 months old
- Had one MMR vaccine and another dose of measles vaccine
- Are established to be resistant to measles, mumps, and rubella after a blood test

The vaccine should not be taken by:

- Girls that are pregnant or intend to become pregnant soon
- People who have a severe allergy to gelatin or neomycin, an antibiotic

Anyone whose immune system could be jeopardized with a treatment or condition for a state should ask their physician if they ought to get the vaccine. Scientists have found no signs of a hyperlink, although there's been a concern with the alleged connection between the MMR vaccines and the probability of autism. The CDC points out that during an epidemic of measles from the U. S. between 1989 and 1991, 90 percent of mortal cases were between those without a history of vaccination.

They state:

- "The main reason for the measles resurgence of 1989-1991 was reduced vaccination policy"

The CDC encourages individuals to have their kids vaccinated to avoid the probability of an outbreak and the spread of measles.

Chapter 6: Tuberculosis (1882-2015)

Tuberculosis (TB) is an infectious illness usually due to Mycobacterium tuberculosis (MTB) bacteria. Tuberculosis damages the lungs, but can also damage other areas of the human body. Most diseases show no symptoms, in which case it is known as latent tuberculosis. Approximately 10% of latent infections progress to active disease which, if left untreated, kills about half of those affected. The signs of TB are cough with mucus, fever, night sweats, and weight reduction. It was called "consumption" because of the weight reduction. Infection of different organs can lead to a range of symptoms. Tuberculosis is spread through the air when individuals sneeze, or who have active TB in their lungs and cough or sneeze. The illness is not spread by people with latent TB. The disease occurs more frequently in people who smoke and in people with HIV/AIDS. Identification of TB relies on microscopic examination and culture, in addition to chest X-rays of human body fluids. Identification of latent TB trusts in the tuberculin skin test (TST) or blood tests. Prevention of TB entails screening those at elevated risk, early detection and treatment of all cases, and vaccination using the bacillus Calmette-Guérin (BCG) vaccine. People at risk include office, family, and social contacts of individuals with TB. Treatment requires the use of antibiotics during an extended time period. Antibiotic resistance is an increasing problem with raising rates of numerous bronchial tuberculosis (MDR-TB) and broadly drug-resistant tuberculosis (XDR-TB). As of 2018 one quarter of the planet's population is supposed to have a latent infection with TB. New infections occur in approximately 1 percent of the populace every year. In 2018, there have been more than 10 million cases of active TB which led to 1.5 million deaths. This makes it the primary cause of death in the infectious illness. More than 95 percent of deaths occurred in developing countries and more than 50 percent in India, China, Indonesia, Pakistan, and the Philippines. The amount of new cases annually has decreased since 2000. Approximately 80 percent of individuals in African and Asian nations test positive and 10 percent of men and women in the USA population test positive by the tuberculin test. Tuberculosis has been present in humans since ancient times.

TB Disease (Latent TB)

Someone can have TB germs in their body rather than expand symptoms. In the majority people, the immune structure can hold the bacteria so that they do not replicate and cause disease. In cases like this, someone will have TB disease but not active disease. Doctors refer to this TB. Someone may be unaware they have the disease and might never experience symptoms. There's also no danger of passing a latent disease to someone else. But treatment is still required by an individual with latent TB. The CDC estimates that as many as 13 million people in the U. S. have latent TB.

TB Disease (Active TB)

Your system may be not able to include TB bacteria. This is more common if the immune system is weakened as a result of the use of medications or disease. While this occurs, the bacteria leading to active TB can replicate and cause symptoms. The disease can be spread by Individuals with active TB. Without intervention, TB becomes active in 5-10 percent of individuals with the disease. In about 50 percent of those folks, the development happens within two-five decades of getting the infection, according to the CDC.

The risk of growing Active TB is greater in:

- Anyone with a weakened immune system
- Anybody who developed the disease from the previous 2-5 years
- Elderly adults and young kids
- Individuals who use Injectable recreational medications
- Individuals who have not received proper Treatment for TB previously

Early Warning Signals

Someone should visit a Doctor if they encounter:

- A cough that is persistent, lasting three or more months
- Phlegm, which may have blood inside when they cough

- A reduction of weight and appetite
- An overall sense of exhaustion
- Swelling in the throat
- A fever
- Night sweats
- Chest pain

Symptoms

- **Latent TB:** An individual with latent TB will have no signs, and no harm will reveal on a torso X-ray. But skin prick test or a blood test will imply they have TB disease.
- **Active TB:** An individual with active TB disease may encounter a cough that produces phlegm, fatigue, a fever, chills, and a reduction of weight and appetite. They're also able to spontaneously go away and go back, although symptoms worsen over time.

Beyond The Lungs

TB usually affects the lungs, even though symptoms may grow in additional areas of the body. This is more prevalent in people with weakened immune systems.

TB can lead to:

- Persistently swollen lymph nodes, or "swollen glands"

- Abdominal pain
- Joint or bone pain
- Confusion
- A persistent headache
- Infection

Diagnosis

An Individual with latent TB is going to have no signs; however, the disease can appear on tests. Individuals should request a TB test if they:

- Have spent some time with someone that has or is in danger of TB
- Have spent time at a state with high levels of TB
- Work within an environment in which TB might be present

A physician will ask about any symptoms and the personal medical history. They will carry out a physical examination, which entails assessing for swelling in the lymph nodes and listening to the lungs.

Two tests can reveal whether TB germs exist:

- The TB skin test
- The TB blood test

However, these can't signify whether TB is active or latent. To check for active TB disease, the physician may suggest a torso X-ray and a sputum test. Everybody with TB requires treatment, irrespective of whether the disease is latent or active.

Treatment

With early detection and proper antibiotics, TB is treatable.

The Ideal Sort of Antibiotic and duration of Treatment depends on:

- The individual's age and general health
- If they've latent or active TB
- The location of this disease
- If the strain of TB is drug-resistant

Treatment for latent TB may vary. It may entail taking an antibiotic once a week for 12 weeks or every day for 9 months. Treatment for active TB could entail taking medications for 9 weeks to 6 months. When an individual has a drug-resistant strain of TB, the treatment will probably be more complicated. It's crucial to finish the complete course of treatment, even if symptoms go away. If someone stops taking their medication early, some germs can survive and eventually become immune to antibiotics. In cases like this, the individual might go on to create a drug. Based upon the areas of the human body which TB impacts, a physician can prescribe corticosteroids.

Causes

M. tuberculosis germs cause TB. They could spread through the atmosphere in droplets if an individual sneezes, coughs, spits, talks, or laughs. The disease can be transmitted by individuals with active TB. When they've received Treatment for a minimum of two weeks, most individuals with the disease can transmit the bacteria.

Prevention

Ways of preventing TB from infecting others includes:

- Getting a diagnosis and premature Treatment
- Staying away from others until there's not any probability of disease

Sporting a mask, covering the mouth, and repainting chambers

TB Vaccination

In some countries, children get vaccination -- the Bacillus Chalmette--Guérin (BCG) vaccine -- as part of a normal immunization program. But, specialists in the U. S. don't advocate BCG inoculation for many Individuals unless they have a higher risk of TB. A few of the causes include a reduced risk in the nation and a likelihood that the vaccine is going to interfere with any TB skin tests.

Risk Factors

Individuals with weakened immune systems are most likely to develop TB. Listed here are:

HIV

For those who have HIV, physicians consider it an opportunistic disease. This usually means that an individual who has HIV has a greater chance of developing TB and experiencing more severe symptoms than an individual having a healthy immune system. TB can grow to be a complication of HIV. Learn more about complications.

Smoking

Tobacco use and secondhand burn boost the risk of rising TB. These variables make the disease more difficult to treat and more likely to come back after treatment. Avoiding contact and quitting smoking can cut the chance of TB.

Other Ailments

Other health troubles that fail the immune system and may increase the chance of developing TB contain:

- Low body fat
- Substance abuse disorders
- Diabetes
- Silicosis
- Severe kidney disorder
- Head and neck cancer

Additionally, some therapies, like an organ transplant, impede the performance of the immune system. Time in a country could raise the possibility of developing it. In the WHO, use this instrument for information concerning the incidence of TB in nations.

Global Responsibilities Along With The WHO Reaction

On 26 September 2018, the UN conducted its first assembly on TB. It followed the international summit on TB hosted by the government and WHO. The result was a political statement agreed by all UN Member States, where existing obligations into the sustainable progress Goals (SDGs) and WHO's End TB Plan were reaffirmed and new ones included. SDG Target 3.3 comprises finishing the TB outbreak by 2030. The End TB Strategy defines landmarks (such as 2020 and 2025) and targets (such as 2030 and 2035) for reductions in TB cases and deaths. The targets for 2030 are a 90 percent decline in the amount of TB deaths and an 80 percent decrease in the TB incidence rate (new cases per 100, 000 inhabitants per year) in comparison with levels in 2015. The landmarks for 2020 are a decline in the TB prevalence rate along with the amount of TB deaths. The plan contains a 2020 landmark that their families and no TB patients face costs.

The political statement Of the UN high-level assembly included four new international targets:

- Treat 40 million individuals for TB disease from the 5-year interval 2018-2022;
- Reach 30 million people with TB preventive cure to get a latent TB disease at the 5-year interval 2018-2022;
- Mobilize US$ 13 billion yearly to get worldwide access to TB diagnosis, treatment and care from 2022;
- Mobilize at least US$ two billion annually.

The UN was asked by the Secretary-General, with assistance from WHO, to supply a report from 2020 into the General Assembly on national and global advancement since the foundation for an extensive review in a high-level assembly in 2023. The Director-General of WHO was asked to continue to develop a multisectoral liability framework for TB (MAF-TB) and also to make sure its timely execution.

WHO is functioning intimately with countries, partners and civil society in scaling up the TB response. Six core acts are being chased by WHOM to contribute to attaining the targets of the UN high-level assembly political statement, SDGs, End TB Plan, and WHO strategic priorities:

- Providing global leadership to finish TB through plan development, political and multisectoral participation, strengthening liability and review, advocacy, and partnerships, including civil society;
- Shaping the TB research and innovation agenda and stimulating the creation, translation, and dissemination of knowledge
- Setting standards and criteria on TB prevention, care and encouraging and facilitating their execution;
- Creating and encouraging ethical and evidence-based policy choices for TB prevention and maintenance;
- Ensuring the supply of specialized technical assistance to Member States and spouses together with WHO regional and country offices, enhancing alteration, and making sustainable capability;
- Tracking and reporting on the condition of the TB outbreak and advancement in the implementation and financing of the reaction at international, regional, and state levels.

Chapter 7: Leprosy (1873-2014)

Leprosy is a disease Mycobacterium leprae, which causes harm to the skin and the peripheral nervous system. The disease develops gradually (from 6 months to 40 years) and also leads to skin lesions and deformities, most frequently affecting the cooler areas within the body (as an instance, eyes, nose, earlobes, palms, feet, and testicles). Skin lesions and deformities can be extremely disfiguring and are why people considered infected become outcasts in several civilizations. Though human-to-human transmission is the principal source of disease, three additional species may carry and (infrequently) move M. leprae to individuals: chimpanzees, mangabey monkeys, and nine-banded armadillos. The disorder is known as a chronic granulomatous disease, much like tuberculosis, since it creates inflammatory nodules (granulomas) from the skin and peripheral nerves over time.

The History Of Leprosy (Hansen's Disease)

Alas, the history of leprosy and its interaction is one of mistake and anguish. The most recent health study indicates that M. leprae has contaminated individuals since as early as 4000 B. C. , although the earliest known written reference to this disorder was discovered on Egyptian papyrus in roughly 1550 B. C. The disorder was recognized in ancient China, Egypt, and India, and there are numerous references to the disorder from the Bible. Many civilizations believed the disorder was a curse or punishment from

103

the gods since they didn't understand that the disease is quite disfiguring, slow to reveal signs and symptoms, and had no known treatment. Thus, priests or sacred men treated leprosy, maybe not physicians. Since the disorder frequently appeared in the household, some folks believed it was hereditary. Other folks noted that when there was no or little contact with infected people, the disease didn't infect other people. Consequently, some civilizations believed infected individuals (and sometimes their near relatives) were "unclean" or "lepers" and ruled, they weren't able to connect with uninfected individuals. Frequently infected individuals had to wear particular garments and ring bells so uninfected men and women could avoid them.

The Romans and the Crusaders introduced the disease into Europe. In 1873, Dr. Hansen found germs in leprosy lesions, implying leprosy had been an infectious disorder, not a hereditary disorder or a punishment from the gods. But many societies still ostracized patients with the illness, and spiritual personnel at assignments cared for people with leprosy. Patients who had leprosy were encouraged or forced to live in seclusion up into the 1940s in the USA (by way of instance, the leper colony on Molokai, Hawaii, which was created by a priest, Father Damien and yet another colony or leprosarium created at Carville, La.) because no successful remedies were offered to individuals at that moment. Due to Hansen's discovery of M. leprae, researchers made attempts to locate treatments (anti-leprosy representatives) that could stop or remove M. leprae. From the early 1900s to about 1940, medical professionals recovered oil from Chaulmoogra nuts and rubbed it on patients' skin. In Carville, 1941, a medication that was sulfone, promin, revealed but demanded shots. Dapsone pills were discovered to work from the 1950s, but shortly (1960s-1970s), M. leprae developed resistance to dapsone. Fortunately, drug trials on the island of Malta in the 1970s showed that a three-drug combination (dapsone, rifampicin Rifadin, and clofazimineLamprene was very effective in killing M. leprae. The World Health Organization (WHO) urged this multi-drug treatment (MDT) in 1981 and stays, with slight alterations, the treatment of choice. MDT, nevertheless, doesn't change the harm done to a person by M. leprae before beginning MDT. At this time, there are many regions (India, East Timor) which the WHO and other agencies (by way of instance, the Leprosy Mission) are working to reduce the number of clinical leprosy cases along with other diseases including rabies and schistosomiasis, which happen in distant regions. Though health researchers aspire to eliminate leprosy such as smallpox, endemic (significance widespread or embedded in a region), leprosy makes whole eradication unlikely. In the U. S., leprosy has happened infrequently but is headquartered in Texas, Louisiana, Hawaii, and the U. S. Virgin Islands by several researchers. Leprosy is frequently termed "Hansen's disease" by most clinicians in an endeavor to get reduce the stigmas attached to some leprosy diagnosis.

What Causes Leprosy?

Leprosy Mycobacterium leprae, rod-shaped slow-growing bacillus, which is an obligate intracellular (only develops inside of particular animal and human cells) bacterium. M. leprae is known as an "acid-fast " bacterium due to its chemical attributes. The blot is a good instance of the staining techniques utilized to look at the organisms. The organisms can't be cultured on artificial media. The bacteria require a very long time to replicate within cells (approximately 12-14 times in comparison with minutes to hours to form many bacteria). The bacteria grow best in 80.9 F-86 F; therefore cooler regions of the body tend to develop the disease. The bacteria grow well in the human body's macrophages (a kind of immune system cell) and Schwann cells (cells which protect and protect neural axons). M. leprae is related to M. tuberculosis (the kind of bacteria which causes tuberculosis) and other Mycobacteria that infect people. They are leprosy-related diseases. Just like malaria, patients with leprosy create anti-endothelial antibodies (antibodies from the lining cells of blood vessels), but the function of the antibodies in such diseases remains under investigation. In 2009, researchers discovered a new Mycobacterium species, M. lepromatosis, which induces diffuse disorder (lepromatous leprosy). Considered among those tropical ailments, this brand new species (based on genetic analysis) emerged in patients situated in Mexico and the Caribbean islands.

The Risk Factors For Leprosy?

Individuals at the highest risk are those who live in the areas where leprosy is endemic (parts of India, China, Japan, Nepal, Egypt, and other areas) and especially those people in constant physical contact with infected people. Additionally, there's some evidence that genetic defects in the immune system might cause certain individuals to become more likely to become infected (area q25 on chromosome 6). Furthermore, those who manage specific animals known to carry out the germs (by way of instance, armadillos, African chimpanzee, sooty mangabey, and cynomolgus macaque) are in danger of getting the germs from the creatures, particularly if they don't wear gloves while handling the creatures.

Leprosy Early Signs And Symptoms

Sadly, symptoms and the signs of leprosy are very subtle and occur gradually (usually over the years). The indicators are much like those that may happen with tetanus, syphilis, and leptospirosis. Listed below are the significant symptoms and signs of leprosy:

- Numbness (one of the initial symptoms)
- Decline of temperature feeling (one of the initial symptoms)
- Touch feeling reduced (one of the initial symptoms)
- Pins and needles senses (one of the initial symptoms)
- Pain (joints)
- Deep pressure sensations have been diminished or lost
- Nerve injury
- Weight reduction
- Blisters and/or migraines

- Ulcers, comparatively painless
- Skin lesions of hyper pigmented macules (flat, light regions of skin which dropped color)
- Eye damage (dryness, decreased blinking)
- Massive ulcerations (later signs and symptoms)
- Hair loss (for example: loss of eyebrows)
- Loss of digits (afterward signs and symptoms)
- Cosmetic disfigurement (as an example, reduction of the nose) (later signs and symptoms)
- **Erythema nodosumleprosum:** tender skin nodules accompanied by other symptoms such as fever, joint pain, neuritis, and edema

This sequence of events starts and proceeds on the cooler regions of the body (for instance, the hands, feet, face, and knees).

How Can Leprosy Spread? Is Leprosy Contagious?

Researchers suggest that M. leprae spreads by droplets or secretions in the upper respiratory tract and rectal mucosa. The disease isn't highly infectious like the influenza. They speculate that infected droplets reach other peoples' nasal passages and begin the infection there. Some researchers suggest the infected droplets can infect others by entering breaks in the skin. M. leprae apparently cannot infect intact skin. Humans get leprosy by animals. Occurrence in creatures makes it hard to eliminate leprosy from sources that are endemic. Medical investigators are exploring avenues of transmission for leprosy. Recent researches have shown that many genes (approximately seven) are correlated with a greater susceptibility to leprosy. Some researchers realize that susceptibility to leprosy could be inheritable. The period for leprosy fluctuates from approximately 6 months to 20 years.

The Remedy For Leprosy

Antibiotics treat nearly all instances (mainly clinically recognized) of leprosy. The antibiotics, their doses, and the amount of time of government derive from classification or the shape of this disease and whether the individual is under clinical supervision. Generally speaking, two antibiotics (dapsone and rifampicin) cure paucibacillary leprosy, whereas multibacillary leprosy is treated using the exact same two and a third antibiotic, clofazimine. Normally practitioners administer the antibiotics for at least 6 to 12 weeks or more to heal the illness. Antibiotics can cure leprosy with very little residual impacts on the individual. Multibacillary leprosy may be kept from progressing, and residing M. leprae could be basically eliminated from the individual with antibiotics, but the harm done before antibiotics are treated is generally not reversible. Lately, the WHO implied that single-dose treatment of patients with just 1 skin lesion using rifampicin, minocycline (Minocin), or ofloxacin (Floxin) is successful. Studies of antibiotics are continuing. Each individual, based upon the standards, has a program to get their treatment, therefore a patient's Treatment schedules should be planned by a clinician knowledgeable concerning that individual's first classification. Drugs have been used by medical practitioners to reduce pain and intense discomfort with leprosy-controlled trials demonstrated no substantial impacts. The function for surgery in treating leprosy happens following a patient completing clinical treatment (antibiotics) with adverse skin smears (no detectable acid-fast bacilli) and is frequently only needed in complex scenarios. Many individuals may be treated by particular clinics. The literature includes home remedies as is true with several ailments. By way of instance, home remedies that are theorized incorporate paste made from the neem plant, Hydrocotyle, and aroma treatment with frankincense. Any home remedies should be discussed with apatient's physician beforehand.

Is It Feasible To Stop Leprosy?

Prevention of contact with droplets from other and nasal secretions from patients with untreated M. leprae infection is now the best means to prevent the disease. Treatment of individuals with antibiotics prevents the person. Because researchers speculate that household members have close proximity, individuals who live with family members are likely to develop the illness. Recent findings indicate susceptibility to the disorder can have a genetic foundation, although leprosy isn't hereditary. Many people have exposures to leprosy throughout the world, but the disease is not highly contagious. Researchers suggest that exposures lead to no disorder, and studies indicate that susceptibility is different, in part.

In the U. S. , there are approximately 200-300 new cases diagnosed annually, with many coming from exposures during overseas travel. Nearly all global cases happen in the tropics or subtropics (by way of instance, Brazil, India, and Indonesia). With treating roughly 14 million cases since 1985, the WHO reports about 500,000 cases globally. There is no vaccine. But, there are reports that using the BCG vaccine independently, the BCG vaccine together with heat-killed M. leprae organisms, along with other preparations might be protective, help clear the disease or maybe shorten treatment. Except for BCG being accessible in a few nations, these preparations aren't readily available. Animals (chimpanzees, mangabey monkeys, and nine-banded armadillos) seldom transfer M. leprae into people. It is not a good idea to manage creatures. These animals are a source of endemic infections.

Chapter 8: Malaria (1880-2018)

Malaria is a serious and tropical disease that spreads through parasites. It kills more than 445,000 individuals per year. Although malaria is wiped from the USA, it's still possible to get the disease if you travel to other areas of the earth. The USA has roughly 1,700 malaria cases each year from travelers and immigrants arriving from countries where malaria is more prevalent. These countries have warmer climates that are hot enough for the malaria parasites and the mosquitoes that carry them to thrive. These areas include Latin America, Southeast Asia, sub-Saharan Africa, and the Middle East. Before you travel, check the site of the CDC. You might need to take pills before, during, and after your trip to reduce your likelihood of contracting it.

Why Malaria Is Harmful

Malaria may cause chills, fever, and flu-like symptoms when not treated quickly, which may be life-threatening. The disorder is caused by Plasmodium parasites, which can be carried by Anopheles mosquitoes. Only female mosquitoes spread malaria parasites. It blows when a mosquito bites a man who has malaria. When the mosquito bites its victim, the parasites are injected inside that individual. Once the parasites enter your body, they travel to your liver, where they multiply. They invade your blood cells, which are important cells in your blood that carry oxygen. The parasites get inside them, lay their eggs, and multiply until the red blood cell bursts. This releases more parasites. As they attack more of your healthy red blood cells, this infection can make you feel very ill.

Kinds Of Malaria

There are five species of Plasmodium parasites that affect humans. Two of these are considered the most harmful:

- **P. falciparum.** This is the most frequent malaria parasite in Africa, and it triggers the many malaria-related deaths on earth. P. falciparum multiplies very fast, causing acute blood loss and obstructed blood vessels.
- **P. vivax.** This is actually the malaria parasite commonly seen out of sub-Saharan Africa, notably in Asia and Latin America. This species may lie dormant, then evolve after the mosquito bite.

Symptoms

Symptoms for malaria start after the mosquito bite. Here are some items to keep in mind, however:

- Because the signs are so similar to cold or flu symptoms, it might be hard to tell what you have at first.
- Malaria symptoms do not always appear within fourteen days, particularly if it's a P. vivax infection.
- People who live in areas with lots of malaria cases may

become partially immune after being exposed to it throughout their lives.

A blood test can confirm if you've got malaria. Together with high fever, shaking chills and sweating, symptoms may include:

- Throwing up or feeling as if you are going to
- Headache
- Diarrhea
- Being quite tired (fatigue)
- Body aches
- Yellow skin (jaundice) from shedding reddish blood cells
- Kidney failure
- Seizure
- Confusion

Malaria can make you enter a coma. Kids with Malaria can get anemia, a condition that occurs when you shed red blood cells. They might have difficulty in breathing. In rare instances they can get cerebral malaria, which causes brain damage.

The Treatment For Malaria

Besides care, the staff needs to choose the proper antimalarial medication (s) to deal with malaria. The selection will depend on several factors, such as

- The particular species of parasite identified,

- The intensity of symptoms, and
- Determination of drug resistance depending on the area.

Physicians will administer the medicine or as an antimalarial based on the above factors.

The most commonly used drugs are

- Chloroquine (Aralen),
- Doxycycline (Vibramycin, Oracea, Adoxa, Atridox),
- Quinine (Qualaquin),
- Mefloquine (Lariam),
- Atovaquone/proguanil (Malarone),
- Artemether/lumefantrine (Coartem), and
- Primaquine phosphate (Primaquine).

Can Malaria Reoccur After Treatment?

P. vivax and P. ovale can clot from the liver and trigger relapsing weeks or months following the treatment. The FDA accepted tafenoquine (Krintafel) as a medicine to prevent relapses of Plasmodium vivax in patients 16 years of age and older. It's a single-dose medicine that will offer a substantial new tool in combating P. vivax malaria relapse, according to investigators.

The Prediction Of Malaria

If recognized and when the antimalarial are Utilized and available, malaria's outlook is quite excellent. Worldwide, malaria is responsible for over 400,000 deaths each year. The vast majority of sufferers are kids from Africa. Death is generally due to insufficient access or treatment. P. falciparum will be the species resulting in the many complications, but also has a higher mortality if untreated. Cerebral malaria, a complication of P. falciparum malaria, has a 20 percent mortality rate even when handled.

Is There A Malaria Vaccine?

There's currently no vaccine to prevent malaria. Because of this diversity of the P., along with the Plasmodium species Falciparum species being the parasite, most attempts are directed toward a P. falciparum vaccine. RTS, S/ASO1 is the most innovative candidate as a vaccine. A phase 3 trial of RTS, S/ASO1 has been finished and the results were printed in 2015. The WHO is currently supporting in the pilot's implementation Nations.

Chapter 9: Yellow Fever (1927-2013)

The History Of Yellow Fever

Yellow fever is a serious disease that is virally transmitted through the bite of infected mosquitoes to humans. Although most cases of yellow fever are light and self-limiting, yellow fever may also be a life-threatening illness, causing hay fever and hepatitis (thus the expression "yellow" in the jaundice it may cause). This viral disease occurs in tropical regions of Africa and South America, and every year there is an estimated 200,000 cases of yellow fever globally, resulting in roughly 30,000 deaths. A rise in the number of cases of yellow fever in the past couple of decades has resulted in campaigns targeted at enhancing general awareness and disease prevention with this re-emerging infectious disorder. Several important yellow fever outbreaks have happened throughout history, with the earliest documented outbreak happening in the Yucatan peninsula during the 17th century. Throughout the late 18th century, a serious yellow fever outbreak struck New England and lots of North American port cities. The town of Philadelphia dropped about one-tenth of its inhabitants throughout the 1793 yellow fever epidemic, inducing many prominent figures in American politics to flee town. The final important yellow fever outbreak in North America happened in New Orleans in 1905. From the late 19th century, Dr. Carlos Finlay, a Cuban doctor, first suggested the concept that a mosquito transmits yellow fever. It wasn't till 1900, with all earlier study from Dr. Finlay as a base, which U. S. Army Major Dr. Walter Reed and his staff demonstrated that mosquitoes, in actuality, transmit yellow fever. This revolutionary notion was instrumental in contributing to the subsequent control of yellow fever in a variety of regions. The virus responsible for yellow fever was afterward isolated from the late 1920s, which breakthrough discovery afterward enabled Max Theiler to create the very first vaccine against yellow fever in the 1930s. This thriving vaccine aided control and removed yellow fever from several nations in Africa and South America throughout the mid-20th century. Regrettably, yellow fever has experienced a massive outbreak of this disease that started in 2017 and has spread to many Brazilian states. This caused the deaths of citizens and travelers. The CDC urges travelers (age 9 weeks and older) to be vaccinated against the illness at least 10 days before arriving in Brazil. Those men and women that are unvaccinated and travel to Brazil should avoid areas where vaccination is recommended (see map below in CDC; many regions of Brazil are contained).

What Causes Yellow Fever?

Fever is caused by a virus. The yellow fever virus is a Genus. After transmission of the virus happens, it spreads through the bloodstream and then reproduces in lymph nodes. This dissemination may affect the bone marrow, spleen, lymph nodes, kidneys, and liver. Irreparable harm to the liver, by way of instance, may result in jaundice and interrupt the human body's blood-clotting mechanism, resulting in the hemorrhagic complications occasionally seen with yellow fever.

Symptoms

People with fever don't develop signs, or the signs are mild. Fever has an incubation period of 3 and 6 days for signs and symptoms to appear after a person is infected. The disease can't spread among people. The illness was spread by parasites only. The principal signs of yellow fever are a higher fever, a slow heartbeat, albuminuria, jaundice, congestion of the face, hemorrhage, or bleeding.

Symptoms and signs are categorized into two phases:

From the first, acute Point, the person may encounter:

- Aching muscles, especially the knees and back
- A high fever
- Dizziness
- Loss of desire
- Nausea
- Shivering or chills
- Vomiting

These symptoms usually disappear within 7 to 10 days. 15% of individuals enter another stage, or toxic stage. The signs are more intense, and they might be life-threatening.

These include:

- Recurring fever
- Abdominal painVomiting, sometimes with blood
- Fatigue, sluggishness, lethargy
- Jaundice, which provides the skin and whites of their eyes a yellowish tinge
- Kidney failure
- Liver failure
- Hemorrhage
- Delirium, seizures, and sometimes coma
- Arrhythmias, or irregular heartbeats
- Bleeding from the nose, mouth, and eyes

Between 20 percent and 50 percent of people who develop toxic stage symptoms die within two weeks. Within 7 to 10 times fever is fatal in about half of all men and women who enter the toxic phase. People who recover don't normally have some organ damage and therefore are immune for life.

The Remedy For Yellow Fever

There's no cure for the fever. Treatment is supportive and aimed at alleviating the symptoms of this illness, for example, fever and pain. As mentioned before, the vast majority of individuals who develop symptoms from yellow fever may undergo a moderate course of illness, which will resolve by itself.

Supportive measures of the disorder, and might incorporate

- Oxygen administration,
- Intravenous fluid management for dehydration,
- Drugs to boost blood pressure in cases of circulatory collapse,
- Transfusion of blood products in most cases of severe bleeding,
- Antibiotics for secondary bacterial diseases,
- Dialysis for kidney failure, and
- Endotracheal intubation (placement of a breathing tube) and mechanical ventilation in cases of respiratory failure.

Steer clear of acetylsalicylic acid (Aspirin) and No steroidal Anti-inflammatory Drugs (NSAIDs) due to the greater chance of bleeding. For the first day or two of sickness, infected people should also be dispersed inside or beneath mosquito netting so as to stop additional mosquito vulnerability, therefore eliminating the prospect of further transmission of this disease.

Vaccination

Anyone traveling into an area should receive the vaccine at least 10 to 14 days prior. Before someone could enter some states may insist on a valid immunization certificate. Vaccine dose supplies 10 or more years' protection, and the individual might be protected for life.

Side effects can comprise:

- Headaches
- Low-grade fevers
- Muscle pain
- Fatigue
- Soreness at the injection site
- In very rare instances, babies and elderly individuals can develop more severe reactions, like encephalitis

The vaccine is regarded as safe for individuals aged between 9 months to 60 years.

The next groups of individuals shouldn't have the vaccination:

- Kids under the age of 9 months at the USA (U. S.), unless the probability of yellow fever is inevitable
- Pregnant women, unless the danger is inevitable
- Breastfeeding moms
- Individuals allergic to eggs
- Individuals with weakened immune systems, unless the probability of yellow fever is unavoidable, such as those with HIV, or individuals receiving chemo treatment and radio treatment

Any individual over 60 years old ought to discuss whether to possess the vaccine with a health care provider. It's necessary for travelers to get the vaccination, to raise their security and prevent spreading the illness to other people. Some immigration authorities won't permit travelers to go into a country. After 30 days, 99% who receive the vaccination have complete protection.

The Side Effects Of The Yellow Fever Vaccine

The yellow fever vaccine could have uncommon but severe side effects. Health care professionals administer the yellow fever vaccine in designated vaccination centers. Health care providers will need to think about the individual's health, their risk of exposure to yellow fever, as well as the management before advocating it. To minimize the risk of serious adverse events, the Centers for Disease Control and Prevention (CDC) provides the next vaccination recommendations:

Contraindications (states where the vaccine shouldn't be granted)

- Allergy to vaccine part
- Age <6 months
- Symptomatic HIV disease or CD4+ T-lymphocytes <200/mm3 (<15% of total in children aged <6 years)
- Thymus disease associated with abnormal immune function

- Primary immune- deficiencies
- Malignant neoplasm's
- Transplantation
- Immunosuppressive and immunomodulatory therapies

Precautions (states for the risks of the vaccine and the disorder needs to be carefully considered)

- Age 6-8 weeks
- Age ≥ 60 years
- Asymptomatic HIV disease and CD4+ T-lymphocytes 200 into 499/mm3 (15%-24% of full in kids elderly <6 years)
- Pregnancy
- Breastfeeding

Individuals who do experience side effects of the Stress vaccine will experience symptoms, such as muscular aches, fever, and headache. Nevertheless, in rare instances, serious adverse events in the yellow fever vaccine may happen involving life-threatening anaphylactic responses, yellow fever vaccine-associated neurologic disease (a disease affecting the nervous system), and yellow fever vaccine-associated viscerotropic disease (a disease involving the internal organs).

Chapter 10: The Black Death:

Plague (1346-1353)

The Black Death, also known as the Pestilence and the Plague, was the most fatal pandemic recorded in human history, resulting in the deaths of up to 75–200 million people in Eurasia and North Africa, peaking in Europe from 1347 to 1351. Plague, the disorder brought on by the bacterium Yersinia pasties, has been the root cause. Y. pestis disease most commonly leads to bubonic plague, but might lead to septicaemic or pneumonic plagues. The Black Death was the next plague outbreak listed, following the Plague of Justinian (542--546). The plague generated societal spiritual and economic upheavals on the course of history. Death originated in East Asia or Central Asia attaining Crimea. From that point, it was probably carried by fleas living on the black rats, which went on Genoese merchant boats, dispersing throughout the Mediterranean Basin and reaching Africa, Western Asia, and the rest of Europe through Constantinople, Sicily, and the Italian Peninsula. Present evidence suggests that after it arrived onshore, the Black Death was in substantial part propagated by individual fleas -- that caused pneumonic plague -- along with the person-to-person contact through aerosols that pneumonic plague empowers, thereby explaining the quick inland spread of this outbreak, which was quicker than could be anticipated if the principal vector was rat bugs resulting from bubonic plague. The Black Death was the next tragedy impacting Europe during the late middle Ages (the very first one being the fantastic Famine) and is estimated to have killed 30 to 60 percent of Europe's inhabitants. From an estimated 475 million to 350 -- 375 million in the 14th century, the jolt could have decreased the entire population in general. There were outbreaks during the late middle ages, and also the shortages of labor enabled peasants to raise their wages. Outbreaks of that plague recurred prior to the 20th century at different locations around the world.

When Did The Black Death Begin?

The Black Death swept through Europe and the Middle East around 1346-1353, however, it might have started from Central Asia's Qinghai Plateau. The span of plague epidemics between the 18th and 14th centuries is referred to as the Second Plague Pandemic. The so-called First Pandemic happened from the sixth through eighth centuries A. D. The Third Pandemic lasted approximately between 1860-1960. The Black Death, Benedictow writes, was "The very first catastrophic wave of epidemics" of this Second Plague Pandemic. They continued to kill 10-20 percent of their population, although a few of those outbreaks during the Second Plague Pandemic were devastating.

How Did The Black Death Impact Europe?

As surprising as it might appear to modern audiences, medieval and early modern individuals took this reduction of people, also grew up with the plague. Scientists and physicians also worked to understand and cure the plague better, especially in terms of preventing its arrival and spread in their communities. Many important developments in the history of medicine and health occurred against this backdrop of plague: the rebirth of dissection, the discovery of the flow of blood vessels, and the evolution of public health actions. It's uncertain why the Second Pandemic finished in Western Europe, although it continued to attack the Ottoman Empire and Russia.

When Did The Black Death Finish?

The Great Plague of London in 1665 was the important outbreak in the plague and England also has seemingly vanished from Germanic and Spanish lands. Marseilles, France's plague, in 1720-1721, is regarded as the major plague epidemic in Western Europe. Some historians assert that public health had improved to stop the spread of anxiety, particularly the efficient and orderly utilization of laws. Others point to evolutionary changes in humans, rodents, or in the bacterium itself, but none of these claims seem to be holding up to recent discoveries in plague genetics. What's apparent is that in the four decades between the Black Death and the disappearance of plague in Europe, physicians worked tirelessly to describe, treat and contain this terrifying disease.

Plague and Its history

Plague is a bacterial illness that's notorious for causing countless deaths because of a pandemic (widespread outbreak) throughout the Middle Ages in Europe, peaking from the 14th century. Many historic references clarify the illness that has been known as the Black Death or even a "pestilence from the atmosphere." The earliest reported plague pandemic started in 541 A.D. and lasted for over 200 decades, killing an estimated 100 million people or more during the Mediterranean basin. The Death forced its way, resulting in the death of 60 percent of the population. The pandemic began in the 19th century in China and spread to areas of the planet in towns. More recently, the World Health Organization reported that an epidemic of plague in Madagascar at November 2014 and again from August through October 30, 2017, using a total of 1,801 confirmed, probable, and suspected cases of plague, such as 127 deaths based on Madagascar caregivers. A number of animals and rodents can be infected with bacteria. The germs contract through bites of insects who have fed on rodents. From managing tissues or fluids from infected animals, humans may develop the disease. Individuals with plague may transmit the disease via coughing droplets to people.

What causes plague?

The bacterium Yersinia pestis causes plague. In the state, rodents are infected by the germs. Plague may be found in several regions of earth; however 95 percent of cases now occur in sub-Saharan and Madagascar, Africa. The World Health Organization claims that involving 1,000-2,000 cases are reported each year but they are estimates. The Y. pestis bacteria are observed from the U.S. in semi-arid regions of the southwest. Rat fleas (Xenopsylla species), which feed from contaminated animals, transmit the bacteria into other creatures. Rabbits, ground squirrels, mice, prairie dogs, chipmunks, voles, and rats are cases of animals that can carry the bacteria. The bacteria are thought to persist in a very low level in populations of those creatures. Fleas, which have bitten on these animals, may bite people and animals, when a high number of wild rodents perish. Cats that are bitten become sick, and they might cough droplets. They might take fleas while dogs that are infected might not look sick. The final urban outbreak of individual cases of flea-borne plague in the U.S. happened from the 1920s. Plague from the U.S. is uncommon now but sometimes occurs in the northwestern part of the nation (like Northern New Mexico, Northern Arizona, and Southern Colorado) where wild rodents could be infected. Between 1900-2017, an average of seven cases of plague occurred annually in the U.S.

Different types of plague

There are 3 basic kinds of plague:

Bubonic plague

The most common form of plague is plague. If an infected flea or bark bites you, it's contracted. You can find the germs. Bubonic plague interrupts your lymphatic system (part of their immune system), inducing inflammation within lymph nodes. Untreated, it may move in the bloodstream (causing septicemic plague) or into the lungs (causing pneumonic plague).

Septicemic plague

If the bacteria multiply there and enter the bloodstream, it is called septicemic plague. Both bubonic and pneumonic plague can result in septicemic plague when they are left untreated.

Pneumonic plague

When the germs spread or infect the lungs, then it is called pneumonic plague. The bacteria from their lungs have been expelled into the atmosphere when coughs plague. Men and women who breathe that air may create this kind.

Signs and symptoms of the plague

Symptoms are generally developed by individuals two to six days. There are:

Bubonic plague symptoms

Symptoms of bubonic plague appear within two. They comprise:

- Fever and chills
- Headache
- Muscle pain
- General weakness
- Infection

You could experience swollen lymph glands. These show up in the groin, armpits, neck, or website of this bite or scrape. The buboes are what provide its title to plague.

Septicemic plague symptoms

Plague symptoms start following exposure, before symptoms appear but plague may cause death. **Symptoms may include:**

- Abdominal pain
- Diarrhea
- Vomiting and nausea
- Fever and chills
- Intense weakness
- Infection (blood might not be able to clot)
- Jolt
- Skin turning black (gangrene)

Pneumonic plague symptoms

Plague symptoms might appear as early as one day after exposure. **These indications include**:

- Difficulty breathing
- Chest pain
- Infection
- Fever
- Headache
- General weakness
- Bloody sputum (saliva and pus or mucus in the lungs)

How plague spreads

People usually get plague throughout the bite of insects who have fed on animals like prairie dogs, and mice, rabbits, rats, squirrels, chipmunks. It may also be spread through contact or simply by ingesting an infected animal. Plague may also spread through bites or scratches of cats. It is uncommon for shock or plague to spread to another.

Incubation period for plague

Signs and symptoms of anxiety develop between two and seven times after obtaining the Yersinia pestis disease, though they may appear after 1 day in most cases of exposure.

Treatment for plague

Antibiotics are effective in curing migraines. Examples of antibiotics which may be utilized include ciprofloxacin (Cipro, Cipro XR, Proquin XR), streptomycin, gentamicin (Garamycin), and doxycycline (Vibramycin, Oracea, Adoxa, Atridox). Individuals with plague might require treatment, such as oxygen, respiratory assistance, and drugs to keep blood pressure. Patients with pneumonic plague has to be dispersed to prevent spreading the disease.

Might it be feasible to stop plague? Can there be a plague vaccine?

There's no vaccine. It is possible to lower the odds of contracting plague by rodent-proofing, or diminishing rodent habitat regions around the house, preventing contact with wild rodents, and wearing gloves while handling carcasses of possibly infected animals. Use repellent for clothing and skin while outside or in areas. Whilst permethrin could be applied to clothes, repellent could be implemented to clothes or skin. Use flea-control goods in your pets, and when pets have been permitted to roam free in plague-endemic regions (including the southwestern U.S.), don't enable them to sleep on the mattress; this is going to reduce the odds of transmitting possibly infected fleas. Prophylactic antibiotics should be administered to people with exposure or for people who have come in contact with body fluids or contaminated tissue.

Could plague be utilized as a weapon?

In reality, Yersinia pestis has a history of being used for bioterrorism. Examples are falling fleas and catapulting of corpses over town walls.

Social and Economic Effects of the Plague

The plague had substantial scale financial and societal consequences, a lot of which can be listed in the Decameron's debut. People fled cities, abandoned their family and friends, and closed off from the entire world. Rites ceased entirely or became, and work stopped being done. Some believed that the anger of God descended upon man, fought with the jolt. Some believed they ought to follow the maxim,"Eat, drink, and be merry, for tomorrow you will die." An upheaval underwent by the society to an extent generally seen in conditions like carnival. Faith in faith diminished following the jolt, both due to the passing of a number of the clergy and due to prayer's collapse to stop death and illness. The market failed intense and abrupt inflation. As it had been so hard (and dangerous) to secure goods through transaction and also to make them, the costs of the goods produced locally and those stolen from afar surfaced. The requirement for people was so large that the holdings jeopardized. Serfs were tied to a single master; when the property was left by one, they would be immediately hired by another lord. Keep them and so the lords needed to make changes to make the scenario more rewarding for your peasants. Generally, wages outpaced the quality of living, as well as prices were increased. As a result of the start of blurring distinctions that were financial, distinctions that were societal sharpened. So as to highlight the societal status of the man the styles of the nobility became extravagant. If the aristocracy tried to withstand the changes caused by the 22, the peasants became more permitted, and revolted. In 1358, northern France's peasantry rioted, and in 1378 disenfranchised members.

Chapter 11: American Polio Epidemic (1916)

1916 New York City Polio Outbreak

The 1916 New York City polio outbreak was an outbreak of Polio ultimately infecting several million individuals, and killing more than two million in New York City, primarily from the borough of Brooklyn. The outbreak was formally declared in June 1916, and also a distinctive area force was built under the jurisdiction of Dr. Simon R. Blatteis of their New York City Health Department's Bureau of Preventable Diseases, using broad authority to quarantine those infected by polio and routine hygiene steps thought to impede the transmission of this disease. Polio was a poorly understood disease in this age, and official attempts to stem its spread consisted mostly of quarantines, the close of public areas, and using chemical disinfectants to cleanse regions where the disease was present. Polio clinics were created at different locations in town for quarantine and the treatment of sufferers. Additionally, steps or many treatments were attempted by the population, while actions fell silent. The epidemic subsided together with the origin remaining a puzzle in the winter season.

Progress Of This Outbreak

On Saturday, June 17, 1916, a formal statement of this presence of the polio disease outbreak was created in Brooklyn. Within the course of this year, there have been more than 27,000 cases and more than 6,000 deaths because of polio in the USA, with over 2,000 deaths in New York City alone. According to the figures published by the New York City Department of Health, by June 1916 there have been 114 confirmed cases of infantile paralysis in Brooklyn, nearly all of them in the older South Brooklyn section. The outbreak appeared to be restricted to young children and babies, less than 10 percent of those cases. The Department of Health said that a careful evaluation had failed to substantiate the opinion that the colleges had a talk in spreading the illness, pointing out that over 90 percent of their kids were under the normal school age. The instances weren't restricted or even more widespread in any 1 school district, which they weren't in any way restricted to kids in precisely the exact same classroom. On June 26, 1916, the Department of Health issued a decision noting 37 added cases of infantile paralysis reported on the Department of Health, creating a total to date of 183 cases in Brooklyn. A study of this situation suggested that the illness has been spreading in a southerly direction and has been invading the Parkville section, to the east of Bay Ridge, Brooklyn. From the week preceding that report, 12 deaths have been reported by anterior poliomyelitis (infantile paralysis) from the Greater City, eleven occurring in Brooklyn, nearly as numerous as happened in the whole city throughout the calendar year 1915, when 13 deaths from this disease were reported for the whole year at the Greater City. The twelfth situation was reported in Staten Island on the Department. It was situated within a district. On June 28, 1916, another 23 cases were reported, bringing the total in Brooklyn to 206 cases. On July 1, 1916, 53 new cases and 12 deaths were reported in New York City, creating a total of 59 deaths since the outbreak of this epidemic. Both disorders and deaths afterward continued to rise on a daily basis during the month of July, peaking in early August, by which time the entire number of instances was in the thousands, and also the number of deaths had been over one million. The disease started a gradual decline for much of the rest of the year.

Symptoms And Transmission Of Polio

Polio is an infectious illness that sent and is caused by a virus. Among the acute signs of polio are migraines, as well as the disorder known as "infantile paralysis." The title poliomyelitis consists of Greek and contrasts to grey (polio) marrow (myelon), which describes the tissue in the middle of the spinal cord, which when influenced causes paralysis. Limbs like legs or arms waste away through the years that are the cause of kid legs being related to the disease polio. Permanent paralysis luckily happens in only 0.5 percent of infections. Nearly all infections (72 percent) don't lead to some indicators. Approximately a quarter of cases (24 percent) cause "abortive" poliomyelitis that contributes to nonspecific symptoms for a couple of days, including a fever or a cold, and 1-5% of cases contribute to "non-paralytic aseptic meningitis," where the individual suffers from rigid limbs for up to ten days. The poliovirus is transmitted through the route and is located among people. To put it differently, drinking water that's been contaminated by the stool of an individual mainly transmits polio. The virus spreads particularly, such as when folks defecate in the open, in terms of poor sanitation, or don't filter their water. That the virus could only live in people (and no other creatures) makes it feasible to completely eliminate the disease in the entire world -- whether it had been a virus using an animal host like flu (birds) or tuberculosis (cows) that sometimes mutates to attack individuals, polio could only ever be manipulated but not eradicated. Its incubation period around ten times and three-fourths of ailments not showing any outward symptoms makes polio hard to monitor without being discovered. Since single identified instances may signal bigger outbreaks, the WHO urges to deal with these cases as a public health crisis when just 1 child is diagnosed with a wild, endemic polio disease in a nation that was formerly declared polio-free.

The Vaccine Against Polio

The Development Of The Polio Vaccine

What altered the background of polio was that the Development of a vaccine. US President Franklin D. Roosevelt himself was diagnosed with polio, bound to a wheelchair for the remainder of his life. While this might have been a misdiagnosis at Roosevelt's case, it was crucial for Infantile Paralysis. The Non-profit company soon became famous as "The March of Dimes Foundation", speaking about polio victims' inability and successfully assembled a number of contributions for vaccine research and its own 'Iron Lung' Distribution program. Years of research went into developing an effective vaccine. The graph shows the growth in scientific books from the 1950s on polio. The physician and virologist Jonas Salk put an embryo ahead and the base rolled out a trial of the Salk vaccine. Millions of kids in 44 US states obtained the vaccine or a placebo taken at. 20 Salk's manager Thomas Francis insisted to present a control group trial layout, and therefore paved the way which has become a method in social and medical science studies in the decades. Contributions supported the base from the people, who collected quarters, dimes, and dollars for years in the expectation of study discovering a means against polio. Oshinsky (2005) reports that the base received contributions from two-thirds (a survey claims). On April 12, 1955, the anniversary of Francis, Francis announced that Salk's vaccine was effective and potent in preventing polio. Within two weeks, the US Public Health Service issued a manufacturing permit immunization program. The conference was live-broadcasted to doctors throughout the nation who'd gathered to see the statement. Countless Americans received the information on the radio in celebration of the information.

Vaccine-Induced Polio

Unfortunately, it is likely the live Poliovirus that is employed from the oral polio vaccine (OPV) mutates and thus regains its "neurovirulence." Happily, it occurs extremely rarely (more below), however, it usually means that recipients of this OPV may develop the paralytic symptoms in the vaccine.

There exist two types of all vaccine-induced polio, VAPP and CVDPV:

- If the mutation is impulsive, one describes Vaccine-Associated Paralytic Polio (VAPP) that is not infectious. It estimated that it happens once every 2.7 million doses of OPV.

- The virus may change to resemble the kind of poliovirus if the mutation occurs by transmitting one of the communities over the course of a minimum of one year. This is called a circulating Vaccine-Derived Poliovirus (CVDPV) and this virus could send through the fecal-oral path to other people. Since 2000, 10 billion doses of OPV distributed globally and just 24 CVDPV outbreaks have happened, counting less than 760 cases.

Since the vaccine virus needs conditions of low Vaccine policy, it is not immunization rates that pose the issue, but rather the vaccine itself. The graph shows the amount of circulating Vaccine-Derived Poliovirus (CVDPV) outbreaks between 2000 and May 2016. More than 90 percent of those viruses were a version of this virus that was eradicated in 1999, of serotype 2. Hence, the Global Polio Eradication Initiative changed in an OPV that protects against three serotypes to one, which just protects against serotypes 1 and 3,and this has resulted in a remarkable reduction in vaccine-derived polioviruses. Further below, in part II the advantages of eradicating polio, we show that as 1988 16 million cases of paralytic polio were prevented due to the Global Polio Eradication Initiative's (GPEI) vaccination attempts. Moreover, the initiative has announced that its aim is to switch into the inactivated poliovirus vaccine (IPV), an upgraded version of the Salk vaccine, which can be administered by injection and doesn't bear the danger of vaccine-derived polio strands.

The Amount Of Projected Polio Cases By World Area

From the 1980s more than 350,000 individuals endured polio cases in 2016. The planet saw 20-times as paralytic polio cases every day. The instances are displayed for each of the six WHO world areas and you will be able to alter the perspective from absolute to relative amounts of polio cases by clicking "Relative" in the bottom left of this picture. In the 1980s, between 50 percent and 75 percent of estimated cases happened from the South-East Asia area, this area has not listed one instance after 2011 and has licensed to be polio-free in 2014. This information on the total quantity of polio cases relies on the number of polio cases that were paralytic that documented. Our estimations of the entire amount follow the methodology by Tebbens et al. (2011) 36, which estimates widespread underreporting -- notably in earlier phases -- of polio is then corrects the number of paralytic polio cases to reach the projected true number of instances. For many nations, Tebbens et al. use a correction factor of 7, meaning that they multiply the amount of documented paralytic polio cases with seven to arrive in the real amount of paralytic polio cases per state. We discuss the way we implemented the method of Tebbens et al. (2011) and expanded their research to 2016 and for many nations in the world in a distinct document here. The World Health Organization is based on a method when estimating the number of instances. This visualization by the WHO contrasts the amount of documented cases with the number of projected cases and arrives in quite similar quotes to ours, together with all the estimated global number of paralytic polio cases being over 400,000 from the 1980s.

Chapter 12: AIDS Pandemic And Epidemic (1981-Present Day)

The AIDS epidemic, due to HIV (Human Immunodeficiency Virus), found its way into the United States as early as 1960, but had been noticed after doctors found clusters of Kaposi's sarcoma and pneumocystis pneumonia in homosexual guys in Los Angeles, New York, and San Francisco in 1981. Remedy of HIV/AIDS is through a "drug cocktail" of antiretroviral medications, and education plans to aid people to avoid disease. Originally, infected overseas nationals have turned back in the U. S. boundary to help prevent further infections. The amount of all U. S. deaths from AIDS has declined sharply since the first years of this disease's demonstration domestically. In the USA around 2016, 1.1 million people aged over 13 dwelt with an HIV infection, of which 14 percent were unaware of the disease. Gay and bisexual men, African Americans, and Latinos stay disproportionately influenced by HIV/AIDS from the U. S.

HIV

The human immunodeficiency virus, or HIV, attacks the immune system, especially CD4 cells (or T cells). The virus transmits via bodily fluids like anal fluids, semen, vaginal fluids, blood, and breast milk. Historically, HIV has spread through unprotected intercourse or the sharing of needles for drug use. Over the years,

HIV can ruin many CD4 cells, which the body cannot fight infections and ailments, finally resulting in the most acute kind of an HIV disease: acquired immunodeficiency syndrome, or AIDS. Someone with AIDS is vulnerable to illnesses, such as pneumonia and cancer. An individual with HIV who receives treatment can live quite long even though there is absolutely no cure for HIV or AIDS. In a 2019 study, it was revealed that treaments can stop the spread of HIV.

Where Did Aids Come From?

Scientists have tracked the source of HIV back to chimpanzees and simian immunodeficiency virus (SIV), an HIV-like virus that attacks the immune system of reptiles and apes. In 1999, researchers discovered a breed of chimpanzee SIV named SIVcpz that was almost equal to HIV. Chimps, the scientist afterward found, search and consume two species of reptiles: red-capped mangabeys and larger spot-nosed monkeys, which take and infect the chimps using 2 strains of SIV. Both breeds unite to form SIVCPZ, which may disperse between humans and chimpanzees. SIVCPZ jumped to people when predators in Africa ate contaminated chimps, or so the chimps' infected blood got in the wounds or cuts of predators. Researchers consider the very first transmission of SIV to HIV in people, who then resulted in the international pandemic that happened in 1920 in Kinshasa, the capital and biggest city in the Democratic Republic of Congo. The virus spread could have spread out of Kinshasa along infrastructure routes (roads, railways, and rivers) through migrants and the sex trade. From the 1960s, HIV spread from Africa to Haiti, and the Caribbean when Haitian professionals at the Democratic Republic of Congo returned home. The virus went ahead from the Caribbean to New York City 1970, and then later to San Francisco. Traveling from the USA helped the virus spread.

The Aids Epidemic Arises

Even though HIV arrived around 1970 in the USA, it did not come to public attention until the 1980s. Back in 1981, the Centers for Disease Control and Prevention (CDC) released a report about five previously healthy gay men getting infected with Pneumocystis disease, brought on by the benign fungus Pneumocystis jirovecii. This sort of disease, the CDC noted, never affects individuals with uncompromised resistant systems. The New York Times printed an alarming article about the new immune system disease, which, at the time, had influenced 335 individuals, killing 136 of these. Since the disorder seemed to influence mostly gay men, officials originally called it gay-related immune deficiency, or GRID. Although the CDC found all significant paths of this disease's transmission – and that female spouses of AIDS-positive men might be infected – in 1983, the people considered AIDS a homosexual disease. It called the "gay plague" for several years afterward. Back in September of 1982, the CDC used the term AIDS to describe the disorder for the first time. By the end of the year, AIDS had been reported in many nations.

The HIV Evaluation Arrives

Back in 1984, the origin found by researchers of AIDS – the HIV virus – along with the Food and Drug Administration (FDA) accredited the very first business blood test for HIV in 1985. A lot of tests can detect it now. The evaluations could be tested using saliva, blood, or urine, even although the blood tests detect HIV earlier after exposure because of high degrees of antibodies. In 1985, actor Rock Hudson became the first high-profile fatality from AIDS. In fear of HIV, which makes it into blood banks, the FDA also enacted legislation that prohibits gay men from donating blood. The FDA would update its principles in 2015, allowing homosexual men to donate blood when they have been celibate for a year, even though blood banks regularly check blood for HIV. From the end of 1985, there have been more than 20,000 reported cases of AIDS, together with a minimum of one instance in each area of the planet.

AZT Made

One of the first drugs for HIV, Azidothymidine (AZT), became accessible in 1987. Numerous different medicines for HIV are available and therefore used together in what is called antiretroviral Treatment (ART) or highly active antiretroviral treatment (HAART). The regimes run by preventing the virus from multiplying, giving the immune system an opportunity to recuperate and fight infections and HIV-related cancers. The treatment can also help reduce the possibility of HIV transmission from the mother to the child during pregnancy. In 1988, the World Health Organization (WHO)announced December 1st to function as World AIDS Day. From the close of the decade, there have been 100,000 reported cases of AIDS from the USA, and WHO estimated 400,000 AIDS cases globally.

HIV/AIDS From The 1990s And 2000s

In 1991, the ribbon became a Global symbol of AIDS awareness. In that year, basketball player Magic Johnson announced he had HIV, helping further bring awareness to this problem and dispel the stereotype of it being a homosexual disease. Shortly afterward, Freddie Mercury – lead singer of this group Queen – declared he had AIDS and died a day after. In 1994, the FDA approved the first oral (and non-blood) HIV test. It accepted the urine test along with the home testing kit. AIDS-related deaths and hospitalizations in developed nations started to decrease sharply in 1995 due to new drugs and the introduction of HAART. However, by 1999, AIDS was the fourth most worthy cause of death in the world and the primary cause of death in Africa.

Medical Treatment

Good improvement made in the U. S. after the introduction of three-drug anti-HIV remedies ("cocktails") that formed antiretroviral drugs. Deaths quickly reduced, using a modest but welcome decline in the annual rate of new HIV infections.

Impact On Girls

- More than 256,500 girls are living with HIV in the U. S.
- Between 2010 and 2015, HIV prevalence among women decreased 21 percent.
- Women of color especially affected, and at 2017, Black women accounted for 6 in 10 (59 percent) of new HIV diagnoses among girls; white girls accounted for 20 percent and Latinas accounted for 16 percent.

Effect On Young People

- Teens and young adults are still at risk, together with those below 35 accounting for 56 percent of new HIV diagnoses in 2017 (those ages 13-24 accounted for 21 percent and people ages 25-34 accounted for 35 percent). 51% most young men and women are infected sexually52%.
- Among young men and women, homosexual and bisexual guys, and minorities affected 53 %
- Perinatal HIV transmission, by an HIV-infected mom to her infant, has diminished considerably from the U. S. because of increased testing attempts among elderly women and ART that could stop mother-to-child transmission.
- A recent poll of young adults (18-30) discovered that HIV

stays an issue for young people, particularly for young people of color.

Effect On Gay And Bisexual Men

- While quotes show that homosexual and bisexual guys comprise only about 2 percent of their U. S. inhabitants, 58 percent of male-to-male sexual contact accounts for most new HIV infections (68 percent in 2015, with another 3 percent happening in homosexual and bisexual men with a history of injection drug use) and many folks living with HIV (56 percent in 2015, with another 5 percent occurring in homosexual and bisexual men with a history of injection drug use).

- Annual infections among homosexual and bisexual guys overall and one of Black gay and bisexual men have remained steady in recent decades. But there were increases among groups of homosexual and bisexual men, such as Latinos and young men 25-34.

- Blacks accounted for the greatest number of new investigations (10,069) among homosexual and bisexual guys in 2017, followed by whites (7,607). Also, according to a recent analysis, black homosexual and bisexual men were discovered to be in a higher chance of being diagnosed with HIV throughout their lifetimes compared with Latino and white homosexual and bisexual guys. 64 percent of young nlack gay and bisexual men are at

148

particular risk. Black homosexual and bisexual men ages 20-29 accounted for 52 percent of new diagnoses.

- A research in 20 major U. S. cities discovered that roughly 1 in 5 (22 percent) of men who have sex with guys is still living with HIV. Also, of these, 1 in 4 are unaware of the disease. Prevalence among Blacks was greater (36 percent) and consciousness of disease was reduced (67 percent), in comparison with men who have sex with males in the analysis total.

Chapter 13: H1N1 Swine Flu Outbreak (2009-2010)

2009 Swine Flu Pandemic

The pandemic has been an influenza pandemic that lasted for approximately 20 weeks, from January 2009 to August 2010, and the second of those two pandemics between the H1N1 flu virus (the first being the 1918-1920 Spanish influenza pandemic), albeit a fresh breed. First clarified in April 2009, the virus seemed to be a new breed of H1N1, which led from a prior triple reassortment of bird, parasitic, and human influenza viruses farther united with a Eurasian pig influenza virus, causing the expression "swine flu." The number of confirmed cases was 1.6 million. But some research estimated that the true number involving asymptomatic and moderate cases was around 700 million to 1.4 billion people – 11 to 21 percent of the worldwide population of 6.8 billion. The value of 700 million is more than the 500 million people estimated to have infected with the influenza pandemic. The amount of all lab-confirmed deaths reported on the WHO is 18,449, although this 2009 H1N1 influenza pandemic estimated to have really caused 284,000 (vary from 150,000 to 575,000) deaths. A follow-up study done in September 2010 revealed that the possibility of critical illness caused by the 2009 H1N1 influenza was not any greater than the annual seasonal influenza. In contrast, the WHO estimates that 250,000 to 500,000 people die from influenza that is seasonal.

Unlike many strains of flu, the Pandemic H1N1/09 virus does not infect adults older than 60 years; this has been an odd characteristic quality of the H1N1 pandemic. Even in previously healthy individuals, a small part develop pneumonia or acute respiratory distress syndrome (ARDS). This typically occurs following the start of influenza symptoms and manifests itself. The pneumonia can be even a bacterial pneumonia or lead viral pneumonia. A November 2009 New England Journal of Medicine article urged that influenza patients whose torso X-ray suggests pneumonia get both antivirals and antibiotics. It is a warning signal if a child appears to be getting better and relapses with fever, since this relapse might be pneumonia.

History

Evaluation of this virus in samples of the divergence from various cases suggested that the virus jumped to humans in 2008, after June, and not later than the end of November. The study also showed the virus was latent in cows for many months ahead of the outbreak, implying a need to boost agricultural surveillance to prevent future outbreaks. In 2009, U. S. agricultural officials theorized, though highlighting that there was no way to prove their theory, that "against the popular premise, the new swine flu pandemic appeared on factory farms in Mexico, in cows in Asia, and afterward traveled to North America in an individual." However, another report by investigators at the Mount Sinai School of Medicine in 2016 discovered the 2009 H1N1 virus probably originated from hens in a really compact area of fundamental México. Initially known as an" epidemic," widespread H1N1 disease was first recognized at the state of Veracruz, Mexico, together with signs that the virus was present for weeks before it was formally known as an "outbreak." The Mexican authorities closed all Mexico City's private and public centers in an effort to contain the spread of this virus. Nonetheless, it continued to spread internationally, and practices in certain regions were overrun by infected men and women. The virus was initially isolated in late April by American and Canadian labs from samples obtained from individuals with influenza in Mexico, Southern California, and Texas. Shortly the oldest known human case tracked to a situation from 9 March 2009 at a 5-year-old boy at La Gloria, Mexico, and a rural city in Veracruz. In late April, the World Health Organization (WHO) announced its first "public health emergency of global concern," or PHEIC. In June, the WHO and the U. S. CDC ceased counting instances and announced the outbreak a pandemic. Despite called "swine flu," the H1N1 influenza virus cannot be distributed by eating pork products; like other flu viruses, it normally contracted by person-to-person transmission through respiratory droplets. Symptoms last 4-6 weeks. Antivirals (oseltamivir or zanamivir) are recommended for people with more severe symptoms or people within an at-risk group. The pandemic started to taper off in November 2009, declining until May 2010. About 10 August 2010, the Director-General of the WHO, Margaret Chan, declared the conclusion of the H1N1 pandemic and stated the H1N1 flu event had transferred to the post-pandemic

152

period. According to WHO data (as of July 2010), the virus had killed more than 18,000 peopleI in April 2009. Nonetheless, they say that the entire mortality (such as deaths unconfirmed or unreported) in the H1N1 strain is "definitely higher." Critics asserted the WHO had exaggerated the threat, spreading "confusion and fear" instead of "immediate data." The WHO started an investigation to find out if it had "fearful individuals." An influenza follow up research conducted in September 2010 discovered that "the chance of the majority of serious complications wasn't raised in children or adults." In August 2011, researchers estimated that the 2009 H1N1 global disease rate was 11 to 21 percent lower than that which previously expected. But by 2012, the study demonstrated that as many as 579,000 individuals might have been killed by the disorder, as only these deaths supported by lab testing were contained from the initial amount. All those deaths happened in Africa and Southeast Asia. Experts, such as the WHO, have consented an estimated the death toll to be 284,500 individuals murdisease than the death toll.

Signs And Symptoms

H1N1 flu's indicators are like those of other Influenzas, and might include fever, cough (a "dry cough"), headache, joint or muscle pain, sore throat, chills, fatigue, and a runny nose. Diarrhea, nausea, and neurological difficulties have been reported. Individuals at a greater risk of acute complications include people over 65, children younger than 5, children with neurodevelopmental conditions, pregnant women (especially during the third trimester), and individuals of any age with underlying medical conditions, such as diabetes, asthma, obesity, heart disease, or a weakened immune system (e. g. , taking immunosuppressive drugs or infected with HIV). More than 70 percent of hospitalizations from the U. S. happen to be individuals with this kind of inherent ailments, according to the CDC. Back in September 2009, the CDC reported that the H1N1 influenza "appears to be carrying a heavier toll on chronically sick children compared to the seasonal influenza." On 8 August 2009, the CDC had received 36 reports of pediatric deaths with related influenza symptoms and laboratory-confirmed pandemic H1N1 from local and state health jurisdictions within the USA, with 22 of those kids having neurodevelopmental conditions like cerebral palsy, muscular dystrophy, or developmental defects. Kids with muscle and nerve problems could be at particularly higher risk for complications since they can't cough hard enough to clear their airways. By 26 April 2009 to 13 February 2010, the CDC had received reports of the deaths of 277 children with laboratory-confirmed 2009 influenza A (H1N1) in America.

Vaccines

19 November 2009 had doses of vaccine administered in 16 nations. A 2009 review from the U. S. National Institutes of Health (NIH) concluded that the 2009 H1N1 vaccine includes a safety profile like that of esophageal disorder. In 2011, research by the US Flu Vaccine Effectiveness Network estimated that the general

effectiveness of pandemic H1N1 vaccines at 56 percent. A CDC study published 28 January 2013 estimated that the Pandemic H1N1 vaccine preserved about 300 lives and averted about a million diseases in the USA. The analysis concluded that had the vaccination program began two weeks before, near 60 percent more cases might have been averted. The research was based on an efficacy in preventing cases, hospitalizations, and deaths of 62 percent for all subgroups except individuals over 65, for whom the efficacy estimated at 43 percent. The potency was based on Asian and European research, and professional opinion. The delay in vaccine management revealed the shortcomings of issues with distribution, in addition to this planet's potential for vaccine-production. Some producers and wealthy nations had concerns about regulations and liability, in addition to the coordination of transporting, storing, and administering vaccines to contribute to poorer states.

Treatment

Numerous methods have advocated helping ease symptoms, such as rest and enough intakes. Over-the-counter pain medications like aspirin and acetaminophen do not kill the virus; they might be practical to lessen symptoms. Aspirin and salicylate products should not be administered to people younger than 16 without any flu-type symptoms due to the risk of developing Reye's syndrome. If the fever is mild, medicine is not suggested. Many men and women recover without attention, though ones with underlying or preexisting medical conditions are more vulnerable to complications and might receive help from added remedies. Individuals in classes must be treated with antivirals (oseltamivir or zanamivir) when possible if they experience influenza symptoms. The groups include kids, pregnant and post-partum women under two years old, and individuals with conditions like respiratory problems. Individuals that are not within an at-risk team who have fast or persistent symptoms must be treated with antivirals. Individuals that have developed pneumonia require antivirals and antibiotics several instances when H1N1-caused disease to develop. Antivirals are helpful and might help improvement if given within two days of the onset of symptoms. In those 48 hours when patients are severely or moderately ill, antivirals may be beneficial. In the case oseltamivir (Tamiflu) is inaccessible or cannot use, Zanamivir (Relenza) advocated as a replacement. Peramivir is an antiviral drug approved in most scenarios where the available techniques of treatment are unavailable or ineffective. To help prevent shortages of those medications, the U. S. CDC advocated oseltamivir for treatment when hospitalized with influenza.

Side Effects

Side effects of both drugs mentioned above for treatment, Zanamivir, and oseltamivir, have proven side effects, such as lightheadedness, loss of desire, chills, nausea, vomiting, and difficulty breathing. Kids reported to be at heightened risk of self-injury and confusion following taking oseltamivir. The WHO cautioned against buying drugs illegally.

Chapter 14: West African Ebola Outbreak (2014-2016)

Western African American Ebola Virus Epidemics

The Western African American Ebola virus epidemic (2013-2016) was that the most widespread outbreak of Ebola virus disease (EVD) in history, causing significant loss of life and socioeconomic disturbance from the area, mainly in Guinea, Liberia and Sierra Leone. The cases were listed in December 2013 and spread from Guinea into neighboring Sierra Leone and Liberia. It caused considerable mortality, together with all the case fatality rate reported that was originally significant, while the rate of hospitalized patients was 57-59 percent. Outbreaks happened in Mali and Nigeria, and diseases of workers happened in Spain and the USA. Additionaly, there were isolated instances that were isolated were listed in Italy, the UK and Senegal. The amount of cases then started to fall slcation of resources. InCurrently May 2016, the World Health Organization (WHO) and variou governments reported that a total of pected instances and 11,323 deaths (39. 5 percent), although the WHO considers that this considerably understates the size of the outbreak. A Pulic Health Emergency of Worldwide Concern was announced and about 29 March 2016, the WHO declared the Public Health Emergency of

Concern Condition of the outbreak. After flare-ups happened, ; tthe final was announced over on 9 June 2016, 42 days after the previous case examined negative on 28 Al 2016 at Monrovia. The epidemic left around 17,000 survivors of this disease, lots of whom report symptoms that were post-recovery termed syndrome severe enough to require clinical attention. Another cause of concern is that the apparent ability of this virus to "hide" at a retrieved survivor's body for an elongated time peand become energetic months or years afterwards, either at the exact same person or within a sexual partner. In December 2016, the WHO declared that a trial of this vaccine that was RVSV-ZEBOV seemed to provide protection against EBOV accountable for its Western Africa outbreak's version. The vaccine is regarded as powerful and is the sole prophylactic that features protection; therefore, 300,000 doses are stockpiled. RVSV-ZEBOV obtained regulatory approval in 2019.

The Signs Of Ebola

Signs of Ebola virus infection include body temperatures, headache, abdominal pain, diarrhea, nausea, and internal and external bleeding, like from feces and gums. It can be tricky to differentiate Ebola from diseases like meningitis, typhoid fever, and malaria. After contracting the illness, symptoms may appear.

Is Ebola Treatable?

There's no proven treatment for the virus. Possible treatments such as blood, immunological, and medication therapies are being improved, and an experimental Ebola vaccine demonstrated tremendously effectiveness in a 2015 trial in Guinea. The Ebola vaccine is used from the Democratic Republic of Congo to provide immunity to individuals at risk for the illness, including households. The vaccine demonstrated effectiveness and is safe, but it isn't licensed for usage.

The Ebola Virus Spread

Ebola is infectious, meaning contact doesn't propagate via the air, although small quantity virus may result in disease. People today become infected from contact with infected animals with the virus by exposure to the bodily fluids of infected men and women, or from eating and butchering meat. The bodies take high concentrations of the virus, which may spread through contact to other people. Supplying safe and dignified burials for individuals is essential in preventing the spread of this illness.

Just How Many People Died During The 2014 Ebola Virus Epidemic?

Throughout the Ebola virus epidemic in West Africa, 11,310 people died, and there have been 28,616 instances that were reported.

2014 -- Initial Major Ebola Outbreak Starts

The virus wasn't well after the outbreak started in 2014 and attained epidemic proportions.

- **March:** Examples of Ebola are reported in Guinea, in Sierra Leone and Liberia.
- **May:** The funeral of a traditional healer in Sierra Leone might have contributed to 365 instances.
- **August:** The World Health Organization (WHO) admits that the outbreak is a "global health issue," warning that 20,000 people could become infected until it is suppressed. Sierra Leone shuts colleges and outlaws meetings.
- **September:** U. S. sends 3,000 military personnel to install 17 therapy centers. U. N. Security Council acknowledges that the outbreak is a danger to global peace and safety.
- **September 19 to 21:** A three-day national lockdown happens in Sierra Leone to identify new instances and disrupt the spread of this illness. While the country's populace was quarantined in their homes, community health workers went door to door, exploring deaths not reported to the authorities and warning families of the hazards of conventional burials, which was an integral element in the spread of this virus.
- **September 30:** Total, there have been 6,574 instances and 3,091 deaths.

- **October 12:** Total increased to 8,997 instances and 4,493 deaths.
- **December 29:** Year-end totals are over 20,000 infections, with 7,900 deaths.

Treatment

No Ebola treatment that is recognized exists. Measures could be taken to enhance a patient's likelihood of success. Ebola symptoms can start as early as two weeks or 21 days. Symptoms usually start with a surprising influenza-like disease characterized by feeling exhausted, and pain in the joints and muscles. Later, symptoms may include nausea, headache, and stomach pain. This can be accompanied by severe vomiting and diarrhoea. In previous outbreaks, it's been noted that some patients bleed externally. Nonetheless, data released in October 2014 revealed that this was a rare symptom from the Western outbreak. Another study published in October 2014 indicated that an individual's genetic makeup can play a significant part in determining how an infected person's body responds to the illness, together with a few infected individuals experiencing no or mild symptoms, while others progress to a very acute stage that includes bleeding. Without fluid replacement, this intense loss of fluids results in dehydration, which then can cause hypovolemic shock – a condition where there is not sufficient blood in your heart to pump throughout the body. When a patient is awake and isn't vomiting, oral rehydration treatment could be instituted, but individuals that are vomiting or so are delirious has to be administered with intravenous (IV) treatment. However, administration of IV fluids is tough in the African atmosphere. Adding an IV needle whilst wearing three pairs of goggles and gloves which might fog up is tough, and once set up, the IV line and site has to be continuously monitored. Without adequate staff to take care of patients, needles might become dislodged or pulled out with a delirious patient. An individual's electrolytes have to be carefully monitored to ascertain correct fluid management, for which most regions didn't have access to the essential laboratory services. Treatment centers were overflowing with patients while others waited to be confessed. Secure burials was tricky due to an abundance of deceased patients. Based on several years of expertise in Africa – and many months working from the current epidemic – MSF chose a traditional strategy. While utilizing IV therapy for as many patients as they could handle, they contended that managed IV therapy wasn't useful and might even kill a patient if not properly handled. They also said they were worried about additional danger to already overworked staff. While experts have analyzed the mortality rates of various treatment settings, and also given the broad differences in factors that influenced results, sufficient information hadn't yet been assembled to create a definitive statement regarding what comprised optimum care from the Western setting. Paul Farmer of Partners in Health, an NGO that as of January 2015 had started to take care of Ebola patients, ardently supported IV treatment for all Ebola patients, saying: "What should the fatality rate is not the virulence of disorder but the recurrence of their medical delivery."

Farmer suggested that each and every treatment Center needs to have a group that specializes in inserting IVs, or even better, peripherally inserted central catheter lines.

Vaccines

Several Ebola vaccines have been developed at the Decade before 2014 and were demonstrated to protect nonhuman primates against disease, but none had been approved for clinical use in humans. In accordance with some 2015 review post, about 15 distinct vaccines have been in pre-clinical phases of development, such as DNA vaccines, virus-like particles and viral vectors. About seven other vaccines were being developed as well. There were just two phase III studies being conducted with two vaccines. In July 2015, researchers announced that a vaccine trial in Guinea was finished that seemed to provide protection. The vaccine, RVSV-ZEBOV, had demonstrated high efficacy in humans, but more conclusive evidence was necessary about its capability to safeguard people through "herd immunity." The vaccine trial used "ring vaccination," a method which was also utilized from the 1970s to eliminate smallpox, where health workers control an epidemic by vaccinating all guessed infected people within the surrounding region. Back in December 2016, the Guinea trial's outcomes have been published announcing that RVSV-ZEBOV was discovered to protect. Following an interval whilst at the group not vaccinated, 23 instances of the almost 6,000 people had contracted Ebola. Along with demonstrating high efficacy among people vaccinated, the trial also revealed that unvaccinated individuals were protected from Ebola virus throughout the ring vaccination approach, termed "herd immunity." The vaccine hasn't had regulatory acceptance, but there are 300,000 doses have been stockpiled. Scientists have discovered the results "very reassuring but there's still a good deal more work to be performed on vaccines for Ebola. " Not yet understood is the period of time a vaccination will be successful and if it is going to prove successful for its Sudan virus instead of just EBOV that is accountable for its Western Africa outbreak.

Economic Effects

Along with this reduction of existence, the epidemic had a number of consequences that are significant. In March 2015, the United Nations Development Group reported due to a drop in commerce, closing of boundaries, flight cancellations, and fall in foreign tourism and investment action triggered by stigma, the outbreak resulted in vast financial implications both at the affected regions and throughout Africa. A September 2014 report from the Financial Times indicated that the effect of this Ebola outbreak could kill more people than the disorder. With respect to Ebola and financial activity in the nation of Liberia, a study found that 15 percent of food companies, 8 percent of construction companies, 8 percent of companies and 30 percent of restaurants had closed as a result of the Ebola outbreak. Montserrado county experienced up to company closing. This signaled a decrease from the Liberian market that Montserrado's county was hit. The capital city

Monrovia endured restaurant and construction unemployment the most while the food and drink sectors suffered. Recuperation in the close of the outbreak, at the market, has been anticipated to be rapid in some industries than others. In the event the decrease in activity dropped, the authors indicated a focus to support the health care system. The World Bank had estimated a reduction of $1. 6 billion in earnings for all three influenced Western African nations united for 2015. In counties affected by the outbreak, the amount of people fell by 24 percent. Montserrado found a decrease. Another study demonstrated that this Ebola outbreak's impact could be felt because of preexisting vulnerability for many years. The consequences were seen in Liberia, like expansions from the mining business' conclusion. Scenarios had put losses that were anticipated in $25 billion. Nonetheless, World Bank estimates were considerably lower, at about 12 percent of the 3 worst hit countries' GDP. The authors went on to say that vulnerability suggested a classification based on factors instead of signs, like food insecurity or lack of physicians, which have been issues and has variables. Regardless of the conclusion of inflows from international donors and war since 2003, Liberia's reconstruction was non-productive and slow. Sanitation facilities, water delivery systems, and electricity endured in Monrovia. Before, the outbreak centers didn't have potable light water or pipes. The authors suggested that shortage of food and other consequences would continue from the inhabitants after the Ebola outbreak had stopped.

Other economic Effects were as follows:

- Back in August 2014, it had been reported that flights had been suspended by airlines. Stores and markets had closed because of travel cordon sanitaire constraints, or even fear of human contact, which led for dealers and producers.

- Pursuits were from affected areas disrupted by movement of people. The FAO warned that the epidemic could undermine food safety and harvests, and that with motion constraints and of the quarantines placed on these, over 1 million people might be food deprived by March 2015. From 29 July, the World Bank had awarded 10,500 tons of maize and rice seed into the 3 hardest-hit nations to assist them with reconstructing their own agricultural systems.

- Tourism was affected by the nations that were affected. Back in April 2014, Nigeria reported that 75 percent of hotel business dropped because of fears of the epidemic. African countries that weren't directly influenced by the virus reported consequences. For instance, in 2015, it had been reported that Gambia's tourism had dropped below 50 percent of its usual business during precisely the exact same period the previous year. Elmina Bay at Ghana had an 80% reduction in US tourism, as well as Kenya, Zimbabwe, Senegal, Zambia, and Tanzania.

- Some mining firms reduced back surgeries, and withdrew all employees' investment that were fresh. In December 2014, it had been noted that African Minerals, the iron ore mining company, had begun its own Sierra Leone operations' shutdown since it ran low on earnings. In

167

March 2015, it had been reported that Sierra Leone had started to diversify on account of the current issues of the country. Back in January 2015, Oxfam Organization suggested a "Marshall Plan" (a reference to the Gigantic plan to reconstruct Europe after World War II) was required so that nations could start to help. The call was repeated in April 2015 when the most-affected African Nations requested for an $8 billion "Marshall Plan" to rebuild their economies. Speaking in the International Monetary Fund and the World Bank (IMF), Liberian president Ellen Johnson Sir leaf said the amount had been required. Sinecure wellbeing systems dropped, investors abandoned our nations, earnings decreased and spending increased."

Conclusion

Most virus pandemics have been caused by influenza (flu) viruses. Flu viruses can vary from season to season and while health professionals are fairly good at predicting the way the virus will alter, sometimes a brand-new virus pops up which does not behave as predicted. That is when a pandemic is most likely to happen because the majority of individuals do not have immunity to the new virus. The deadliest pandemic in history has been that the Spanish influenza of 1918. The virus infected with an estimated one-fifth of the planet's inhabitants and has been responsible for inducing between 20 million and 50 million deaths -- that is an estimated 1 percent to 3 percent mortality rate. The virus did not originate in Spain, but the nation has been the first to report the outbreak, therefore people started calling it that the Spanish influenza (the Spanish believed it began in France and called it the "French influenza"). The 1957-1958 Asian influenza pandemic was triggered with a new strain of flu A virus (H2N2) that arose in East Asia, according to the Centers for Disease Control and Prevention. The virus killed an estimated 1.1 million people globally, which equates to an estimated death rate of 0.019 percent, according to a study published in The Journal of Infectious Diseases. The 1968 Hong Kong influenza pandemic was caused by a new breed of the H3N2 virus, which originated from Southeast Asia. The pandemic made its name because rather than due to where the virus originated. The Hong Kong flu killed an estimated 1 million individuals globally, or about 0.03 percent of the planet's inhabitants, according to the CDC. The H1N1 swine flu pandemic of 2009-2010 was due to a new breed of the exact same virus that caused the Spanish influenza -- the H1N1 virus. The influenza-infected an estimated 700 million to 1.4 million people, which has been much more in absolute terms compared with the Spanish flu. However, the mortality rate was much less, in an estimated 0.01 percent to 0.08 percent, according to an investigation published in the journal The Lancet. Seasonal influenza is a yearlong disease burden throughout the planet and even though the vaccine is successful, deaths in flu-related diseases still happen. The World Health Organization estimates that flu causes 290,000 to 650,000 deaths each year.

Among the deadliest pandemics in human history has been the Black Death, a worldwide epidemic of bubonic plague between the decades of 1346 and 1353. The disorder is caused by the bacterium Yersinia pestis, which also led to the passing of somewhere between 30 to 60 percent of the populace of Europe throughout the mid-14th century, though experts believe the disease originated in Central Asia decades before. The initial cholera pandemic happened in 1817 and originated in Russia, in which 1 million people died, based on history.com. The bacterium was sent to British troops, who transported it into India and finally the rest of the world. The Russian influenza of 1889 is regarded as the first significant influenza pandemic. It probably started in Siberia and Kazakhstan prior to making its way west to Europe and across the Atlantic Ocean to North America and afterward Africa. From the end of 1890, an estimated 360,000 people had died from influenza, based on history.com. HIV, that's the virus which causes AIDS, probably developed to people in West Africa from the 1920s, which has been transferred out of a virus. The virus made its way around the entire world and HIV/AIDS proved to be a pandemic from the late 20th century. An estimated 35 million people have died from the disease since its discovery. Drugs created in the 1990s now enable people with the disorder to undergo a normal life with frequent treatment. Even more reassuring, two individuals weree healed of HIV in 2020. The CDC's definition of a flu outbreak relates to the proportion of deaths in a specific week brought on by pneumonia and influenza. The "epidemic threshold" is a specific percentage over what is deemed normal for this period. The standard amount, or baseline, is mathematically determined based on information in previous flu seasons. Christine Pearson, a spokeswoman for the CDC, warns the definition of a flu outbreak does not apply to other ailments. People who perish are a few of the young children, and individuals with weak immune systems, although millions can sicken. That is not true through the flu pandemics. There are two characteristics of a flu pandemic. The virus is a breed that hasn't infected individuals. It's on a worldwide scale. It's also deadly. "A pandemic is essentially a worldwide outbreak -- an epidemic that spreads into more than 1 continent," states Dan Epstein, a spokesman for the Pan American Health Organization, a regional division of the World Health Organization. There was one in 1957-1958 and in 1968-1969. This 20th century's notorious pandemic influenza was in 1918-1919. An estimated 40 million people died in under a year, and also what made it different from influenza epidemics is that young men and women were killed by it.

THE SPANISH FLU

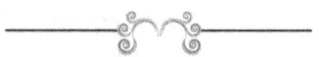

History Of The 1918 Great Influenza Born From
H1N1Virus. The Deadliest Pandemic That The
Human Race Has Faced And Overcome

Introduction

Influenza is a virus that belongs to the Ortho-myxoviridae family. It contains an enveloped virion, which includes a genome made from eight single-stranded negative-sense RNA segments that code for 10 or 11 referred proteins. For example, surface glycoproteins hemagglutinin (HA) and neuraminidase (NA), matrix and ion-channel proteins (M1 and M2), RNA polymerase subunits (PB1, PB2, and PA), nucleoprotein (NP), and nonstructural proteins (NS1 and NS2/NEP), using a few strains encoding another proapoptotic protein, PB1-F2. Reassortment among the flu virus genome segments is visible and it happens frequently. This phenomenon gives rise to mixtures of different subtypes of NA and HA that circulate in host populations. Waterfowl are believed to be the normal reservoirs of the influenza virus nonetheless; the virus is known to infect a lot of different hosts, such as humans, swine, horse, puppy, etc., along with a vast array of avian species. A comprehensive understanding of any pathogen, such as flu virus, necessitates comprehension of how variations in the arrangement of the pathogen genome (genotype) are expressed. This is required as it assists in understanding the differences from the operational qualities of the pathogen (phenotype). It's well-known that flu virus sequences constantly grow by accumulating mutations via a procedure called "genetic drift," where arrangement variants are introduced with the virus's low-fidelity polymerase. These are chosen to maintain significant structural and functional protein traits while trying to evade the host immune system. Comparative genomics research has largely been limited to phylogenetic evaluation of whole-genome sections or statistical institutions of sequence variants at single residue ranks and their impacts on specific phenotypic attributes. Nonetheless, these methods of genomics have limitations. The analysis doesn't consider the effect of genomic residues on the phenotype of attention. Section analysis doesn't highlight the areas responsible for its effect. Additionally, although the ancestry of hereditary variations caused by the cumulative consequences of development can be shown from the phylogenetic tree topology, phenotypic changes arising from convergent evolution aren't shown through phylogenetic tree foliage. Sequence variations may additionally affect virus traits, which might not be subjected to powerful natural selective pressures from the reservoir host. For instance, it could measure the host range specificity of interspecies transmissibility modified with replication virulence and pathogenicity in human and temperature sensitivity. Consequently, a conventional whole-segment phylogenetic analysis might not disclose the many clinically and epidemiologically relevant sequence alterations, because the connections between particular specific phenotypic changes and their underlying genotypic variations might be masked with the intricate global effects of evolutionary selection on the whole viral genome. To deal with these constraints, we've developed a novel way of analyzing the effects of sequence variation on organism phenotypes known as the sequence feature variation form (SFVT) strategy, wherein mixtures of amino acid positions are described as distinct sequence attributes (SFs) according to structural and operational attributes. The amount of sequence variation is ascertained for every SF individually as a pair of version types (VTs) for the SF, which may subsequently be utilized for statistical evaluation of genotype-phenotype associations. The SFVT strategy was described for the institution from the setting of pancreatic.

Chapter - 1 Origin Of The Influenza Pandemic Of 1918-19

The sudden outbreak of the virus in 1918-19 was known as flu Pandemic. It was one of the most severe influenza outbreaks of the 20th century. In terms of absolute numbers of deaths, it was one of the most devastating pandemics in human history. Influenza is caused by a virus that's transmitted from person to person. An outbreak can happen from which the population has no immunity if a new strain of flu virus emerges. The flu pandemic of 1918-19 affected populations to a huge proportion. An influenza virus, known as flu type A subtype H1N1, is currently proven to have become the origin of the intense mortality of the outbreak, which led to an estimated 25 million deaths, even though some researchers have estimated it triggered as many as 40-50 million deaths. The pandemic occurred in 3 waves. The first seemingly originated in ancient March 1918, during World War I. Though it remains unclear at which the virus first surfaced, it rapidly spread through Western Europe, and by July it had spread to Poland. The initial wave of flu was mild. However, a kind of disorder had been known to be caused by it, and this type appeared in August 1918. Pneumonia developed after the initial indications of this influenza. As an instance, at Camp Devens, Massachusetts, U.S., six days after the first case of flu was reported, that there were 6,674 instances. The next wave of the pandemic happened in the next winter, and from the spring that the virus had run its program. In both waves roughly half of the deaths were among 20-40-year-olds, an odd mortality era pattern for flu. Outbreaks of this influenza occurred in almost every inhabited part of the world, first in vents, then dispersing from city to city across the primary transport routes. India is thought to have endured at 12.5 million deaths throughout the pandemic, and also the disease attained distant islands in the South Pacific, including New Zealand and Samoa. Roughly 550,000 people died. Most deaths happened during the third and second waves. Outbreaks of flu happened with virulence in the 1920s.

Epidemic

The epidemic is an incident of disorder that's temporarily high. If the incidence of an epidemic occurs over a large geographical area (e.g., globally), it is known as a pandemic. The rise and fall in the outbreak prevalence of infectious illness are likely to be occurred by the transport of an effective dose of the infectious agent from an infected person to a vulnerable person. Following an outbreak has escalated, the affected server population includes a sufficiently small percentage of susceptible people that reintroduction of this disease won't lead to a new outbreak. Considering that the parasite population can't replicate itself in this kind of bunch population, the host population as a whole is resistant to the epidemic disease, a phenomenon termed herd resistance. After an outbreak, the host population will revert into a state of susceptibility due to (1) the corrosion of human resistance; (2) the elimination of resistant people bypassing, and (3) the influx of vulnerable people by birth. With the years the people as a whole become more vulnerable. The time elapsing between outbreak peaks differs from another and is changeable. From the late 20th century that the definition of the outbreak was extended to include outbreaks of any chronic disease or illness (e.g., cardiovascular disease or obesity). The expression outbreak can be earmarked for illness among human beings; an epidemic of illness among animals aside from man is termed as epizootic.

Influenza

This is also known as a serious viral, grippe, or flu. This disease of the upper or lower respiratory tract is indicated by fever, chills, and a generalized feeling of pain and weakness in the muscles, as well as varying levels of soreness at the head and gut.

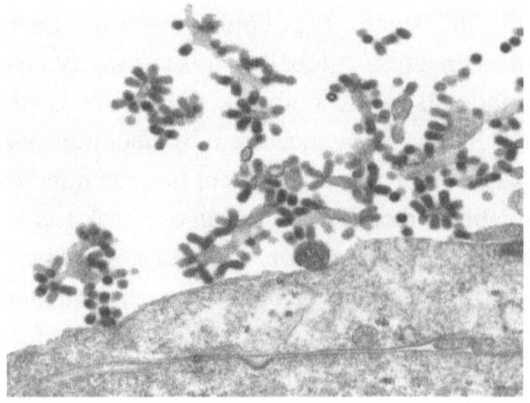

A Sequence Of Influenza Infection

This is any of the numerous sources of influenza viruses from the family Orthomyxoviridae (a group of RNA viruses). Flu viruses have been categorized as types A, B, C, D. These significant types normally produce similar symptoms but are unrelated antigenically, in order that infection with one type confers no resistance against the others. The A viruses trigger the excellent flu epidemics, along with the B germs trigger smaller localized outbreaks. C viruses cause a mild disease. Influenza D viruses aren't known to infect people and have been discovered only in cows. Influenza viruses are classified into subtypes, and subtypes of influenza A and the two influenza B are split into breeds. Subtypes of influenza A are distinguished mainly on the basis of two surface antigens (foreign proteins) --hemagglutinin (H) and neuraminidase (N). Cases of flu subtypes comprise H1N1, H5N1, and H3N2. Strains of influenza strains and B of flu subtypes are further distinguished by variations in the molecular arrangement.

Evolution And Virulence Of Influenza Infection

Between outbreaks, the pandemics viruses undergo continuously, rapid development (a procedure called antigenic drift), which can be powered by mutations in the genes encoding antigen proteins. Gradually, the viruses experience significant evolutionary change by obtaining a new genome section from a different flu virus (antigenic shift), effectively turning into a new subtype. Animals facilitate evolution. If a pig is concurrently infected with distinct influenza viruses, like human, swine, and avian strains, genetic reassortment could happen. This procedure contributes to new strains of influenza A. Recently surfaced flu viruses are inclined to be initially highly infectious and infectious in humans due to the fact that they have novel antigens to the body does not have any ready immune defense (i.e., present antibodies). After an important percentage of people develop resistance through the creation of antibodies capable of preventing the brand-new virus, the infectiousness and virulence of this virus decrease. Although outbreaks of flu viruses are usually most deadly to immature children and the elderly, the casualty rate in people between ages 20 and 40 is occasionally high, though the patients get therapy. This phenomenon is thought to be attributed to the hyper-reaction of their immune system to new strains of the flu virus. Response results in the overproduction of inflammatory chemicals called cytokines. The discharge of excessive quantities of these molecules induces inflammation that is acute. People whose immune systems aren't fully developed (like babies) or are diminished (like the older) can't create such a deadly immune reaction.

Pandemics And Epidemics

Influenza pandemics are estimated to occur on an average of every 50 decades. Epidemics might happen and the flu appears annually sometimes. A pandemic can happen within a matter of weeks, as soon as influenza a virus undergoes an antigenic change. The flu pandemic of 1918-19, the very damaging flu outbreak in history and among the most acute disease pandemics that ever struck, was due to a subtype of influenza called H1N1. In this event, an estimated 25 million individuals world-wide died of this so-called Spanish influenza, which was widely reported in Spain but originated from Kansas, U.S.

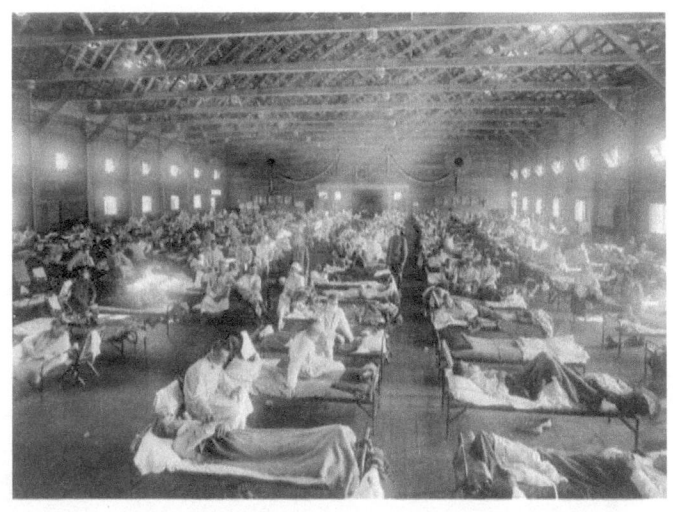

Pandemics of flu have been intense. For example, influenza A subtype H2N2, or the 1957 influenza pandemic, seemingly started in East Asia early in 1957, and by midyear it had circled the world. The outbreak continued to a pandemic amount until roughly the middle of 1958 and caused an estimated 1 million to 2 million deaths globally. Following 10 decades of development that generated yearly epidemics, the 1957 flu vanished in 1968, just to be replaced with a new influenza A subtype, H3N2. This virus is in circulation. The influenza outbreak of 1968 has been the third-largest flu pandemic of the 20th century also led to an estimated 1 million to four million deaths. In 1997 a kind of avian flu, or bird flu, virus awakened among domesticated poultry in Hong Kong, then infected a few individuals, killing a number of them. The exact same virus, H5N1, reappeared in one of the poultry flocks in Southeast Asia through the winter of 2003-04, infecting some individuals fatally. It hasoccasionally reappeared, mostly in wild birds, domestic poultry, and people. A lot of subtypes of bird influenza viruses have been known, such as H7N2, H7N3, and H9N2.

An epidemic of a strain of H1N1 happened in 2009. Initially called swine flu since the virus has been supposed to have been transmitted to humans from pigs; the disease initially broke out in Mexico and subsequently dispersed to the USA. The H1N1 virus that caused the epidemic was found to own genetic material from human, avian, and 2 distinct swine flu viruses. The 2009 H1N1 epidemic was not as fatal as the pandemic of 1918-19. The virus has been spread and highly infectious. The pandemic possibility of this new H1N1 virus has been made apparent to the global community from the World Health Organization (WHO), which broadcasted degree 5 pandemic alerts on April 29, 2009. This prompted the implementation of reduction processes in nations, to treatment centers. Despite all these steps, the virus continued to spread. On June 11, 2009, after an increase in cases in Chile, Australia, and the UK, WHO increased the H1N1 alert level from 5 to 6, which means that the outbreak was formally announced a pandemic. From 2010 individuals in over 209 nations had been affected. It was the first influenza pandemic of the 21st century. In the US, the elevated levels of disease observed through the 2009 pandemic weren't detected again until 2018. Studies have suggested that all the four historical flu pandemics was preceded by a La Niña occasion:a shift in global climate conditions related to cool sea surface temperatures from the Pacific Ocean that some scientists speculate could have shifted the migratory patterns of birds, potentially increasing their interactions with domestic animals and empowering hereditary variety and the growth of new pandemic strains of flu viruses.

Influenza Pandemic Preparedness

Because flu epidemics and pandemics can devastate areas of the planet quickly, WHO monitors flu disease activity on a worldwide scale. This observation is helpful for collecting information that may be employed to prepare vaccines and that may be disseminated to health centers in states where seasonal flu outbreaks will likely happen. Tracking by WHO pandemics plays a significant part in preventing and preparing for epidemics. In case a flu virus appears, WHO adheres to its pandemic preparedness program. This strategy contains six phases of pandemic alert. Phases 1-3, which are the phases in preparedness, are all made to stop or contain outbreaks that were modest. In these early stages, isolated incidences of both animal-to-human transmissions of a flu virus have been detected and supply warning signals that a virus has pandemic potential. Little outbreaks of the disorder may occur resulting, from instances of transmission. Stage 3 signs to states that are affected by the execution of attempts are required to protect against a pandemic. Phases 5 and 4 have been characterized in mitigating the outbreak by urgency. Confirmed human-to-human viral transmission, together with the continual disease in human communities that spread in order that disease transmission between individuals happened in just two states, suggests that a pandemic is imminent. Stage 6 is characterized by illness and transmission of the virus between people. Influenza pandemics happen in waves. Consequently, when illness activity decreases a stage, it might be accompanied by another phase of a high incidence of disease. Because of this, flu pandemics may persist for a period of weeks.

Transmission And Migraines

People of all ages may get affected; however, the prevalence of this disease is one of the adults and kids. Illness is transmitted from person to person in this way as inhalation of droplets leading to coughing and coughing. Since the virus particles gain entry, they ruin and attack the epithelial cells, which line the respiratory tract, bronchial tubes, and trachea. The incubation period of the illness is one or two days, and the symptoms are sudden, with abrupt and different distress, fatigue, and muscular aches. The temperature rises quickly to 38-40 °C (101-104 °F). Acute aches throughout the body and a headache are accompanied by a feeling of rawness in the throat or aggravation. A few times the fever starts to drop, and the individual starts to recover. Feelings of fatigue may be notable and accompany symptoms like coughing and nasal discharge. Complications like pneumonia or pneumonia may occur among individuals and may cause death.

Treatment And Prevention

The antiviral medications rimantadine and amantadine have consequences on instances of influenza between this type A virus. But immunity to these agents has already been detected, thereby decreasing their efficacy. A more recent category of medication, the neuraminidase inhibitors, including oseltamivir (Tamiflu) and zanamivir (Relenza), was released in the late 1990s; those drugs inhibit both the influenza A and B viruses. Aside from this, an intake of fluids, bed rest, and using analgesics is suggested. It's advised as treatment of diseases with aspirin is associated with Reye syndrome, that children and teenagers with the flu not to be given aspirin. Injection of a vaccine may bolster defense against the flu. These germs are produced in chick embryos; preparations that were regular incorporate a number of those a subtypes and the type B flu virus. Security from 1 vaccination lasts annually, and vaccination may be recommended for those people that are vulnerable to flu or whose condition could lead to complications. But immunization in healthy individuals is advised. Advances in the comprehension of influenza and flu technologies enabled the growth of a universal flu vaccine effective at protecting people against a range of flu subtypes.

To be able to prevent bird influenza viruses that are human-infecting out of mutating into more harmful subtypes, public health authorities attempt to restrict the viral "reservoir" in which antigenic change may happen by ordering the destruction of infected poultry flocks.

Pandemic

Pandemic is connected to the geographical area and it might end up affecting a considerable percentage of the planet's inhabitants over the course of many months. Pandemics originate from epidemics, that can be outbreaks of disease restricted to a single portion, like a nation. To ensure that a post-period might be accompanied by another phase of high disease incidence, particularly those involving flu, pandemics happen in waves. Diseases like flu can spread in a matter of days. Numerous factors facilitate the spread of illness, such as an elevated amount of human-to-human transmission of this illness infectiousness of this representative, and way of transport. Diseases that arise in animals cause the vast majority. Therefore, when a new infectious agent or disorder occurs in creatures, surveillance organizations situated within impacted regions are responsible for alerting the World Health Organization (WHO) and also for carefully tracking the behavior of this infectious agent and also the action and spread of this illness. WHO monitors disease action on a worldwide scale by means of a network of surveillance centers found in nations. In the case of flu, WHO has arranged a pandemic preparedness plan that consists of six phases of pandemic alert, summarized as follows:

•   Stage 1: the smallest level of pandemic alert; suggests an influenza virus, possibly just appeared or formerly present, is circulating among creatures. The chance of transmission to humans is reduced.

•   Stage 2: isolated incidences of animal-to-human transmission of this virus have been detected, suggesting that the virus has pandemic potential.

•   Stage 3: characterized by little outbreaks of disorder, normally resulting from several instances of animal-to-human transmission, even though limited capability for human-to-human transmission could be present.

•   Stage 4: supported human-to-human viral transmission which leads to sustained disease in human communities. At this point, containment of the virus is deemed hopeless but there is an inevitable pandemic. The implementation of management methods to prevent additional spread is highlighted in areas of the planet.

•   Stage 5: indicated with human-to-human disease transmission in just two states, signaling that a pandemic is imminent and that supply of stockpiled drugs and implementation of approaches to control the disorder has to be carried out with urgency.

- Stage 6: characterized by sustained and widespread disease transmission among individuals.

When WHO updates a pandemic alert from level 4 to level 5, it functions as a sign to nations to execute the strategies that are suitable. Pandemics of diseases like cholera, plague, and flu have played a part in forming human cultures. Examples of important historic pandemics contain the plague outbreak of the Portuguese Empire in the 6th century CE; the Black Death, that originated in China and spread throughout Europe from the 14th century; along with the flu pandemic of 1918-19, that originated from the U.S. state of Kansas and spread into Europe, Asia, and islands in the South Pacific. Now several diseases happen on a worldwide scale persist in a high degree of incidence, though pandemics are characterized by their incidence on a length of time, and maybe transmitted between individuals. Such ailments represented in contemporary pandemics contain AIDS, caused by HIV (human immunodeficiency virus), which can be transmitted directly between individuals; and malaria, due to parasites in the genus Plasmodium, which can be transferred from one creature to another by mosquitoes, which feed on the blood of infected individuals.

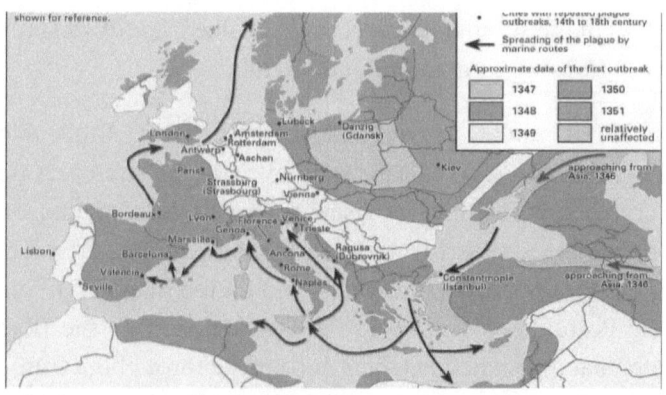

Influenza pandemics are anticipated to occur approximately every 50 decades, although the period in its occurrence has been shorter than that. After 191–9, you will find just two additional flu pandemics: the 1957 Asian flu and the 1968 Hong Kong influenza pandemic. Until about 1958, a pandemic arose that was responsible for over a million deaths. The influenza pandemic happened in 2009 when a subtype of virus spread across areas of the earth. Between March 2009 and mid-January 2010, H1N1 deaths were reported. In March 2020 an outbreak of a Novel coronavirus called severe acute respiratory syndrome coronavirus-2 (SARS-CoV2) was announced by WHO officials. Infection with SARS-CoV2 generated an illness called coronavirus disorder 2019 (COVID-19); the disease was characterized by cough, fever, and shortness of breath. The outbreak started at Wuhan, China in 2019, as soon as a patient with disabilities was admitted to a hospital. In the next few weeks, the number of individuals climbed in ratio, along with the spread of the Wuhan Disease into other areas of China. By 2020, COVID-19 had covered the USA and Europe by travelers. From the time the epidemic was announced, instances of COVID-19 had been discovered worldwide. There were confirmed cases and about 5,000 deaths.

Chapter - 2 The Origin And History Of Spanish Flu

This flu's source has been debated. The Claude Hannoun Pasteur Institute has posited that the virus originated in China, dispersed through troop moves, and from there, to Boston and Kansas, then to Brest, France. Here's a timeline of the Spanish Flu rallied around the globe.

April 1917 - the U.S. enters World War I with 378,000 guys in the armed forces, this can quickly swell to countless guys.

June 1917 - to raise the amount of men, there is a draft created. The military creates each home 25,000 to 55,000 guys, 32 training facilities.

March 1918 - That number increased five-fold a week later. Sporadic cases of the influenza start appearing elsewhere in the U.S., also in Europe and Asia.

April 1918 - that the mention of this influenza seems describing three deaths and 18 cases.

May 1918 - that the U.S. started shipping thousands upon thousands of troops to Europe. Due to the war, censors at Germany, England, France, and the U.S. were blocking news of this epidemic, leaving unbiased Spain to report the disorder. This is how it got the title, the "Spanish Flu." The virus spreads from Europe into North America, Asia, Africa, Brazil, islands in the South Pacific, as well as indigenous tribes living in the Arctic Circle.

September 1918 - another wave of this virus emerges, which has a higher fatality rate than the previous wave. It evolved in an Army facility, also in a Navy facility in Boston just outside the city.

This tide is responsible for the majority of the deaths in the virus, with 12,000 people dying from the U.S. through September. The New York City Board of Health required that cases of influenza be reported and patients are isolated, either in home or in a hospital. To get a Liberty Bonds parade, 200,000 people collect back in Philadelphia, and day's 635 cases of the flu are reported. Theaters, churches, and the town dictate schools were closed.

October 1918 - 195,000 Americans die of the flu in this month. There's a shortage of nurses since most are currently serving. The American Red Cross Chicago Chapter issues a call for volunteers to nurse the ill. Colleges and film theaters close, and public gatherings are prohibited by them. Legislation in Chicago drops by 43 percent. Is made to put away corpses and also a secondhand automobile maker requires packing crates to be utilized as coffins. San Francisco urges that face masks are worn by of its citizens out in people, and in NYC, shipbuilding is down by 40 percent because of absenteeism.

November 1918 - Soldiers are brought cases of the influenza, and back home by the conclusion of the war. Signals are placed by officials at Salt Lake City. In France, the armistice is signed on November 11, 1918, ending WWI. U.S. President Woodrow Wilson collapses after coming down with the flu.

January 1919 - a wave of the virus emerges, killing a lot people. Between January 1st and the fifth, 1,800 influenza cases that are new are experienced by San Francisco, and 101 people perish. New York City reports 706 cases and 67 deaths.

August 1919 - the Influenza pandemic comes to a conclusion because people who have been infected perished or developed resistance.

March 1997 - onMarch 21st, 1997, an article is published in Science Magazine. Researchers at the Armed Forces Institute of Pathology examined lung tissue obtained by a soldier that died in 1918 of this influenza. They conclude that although the influenza virus is exceptional, that, "The hemagglutinin receptor matches closest to swine flu viruses, demonstrating that this virus came to individuals through pigs."

February 2004 - Researchers at the Scripps Institute in La Jolla, California and in England's Medical Research Council conclude that the 1918 virus could have jumped directly from birds to people, bypassing dinosaurs entirely. This may explain the virulence of this disease.

October 2005 - Scientists in the Armed Forces Institute of Pathology order the whole genome of this virus by analyzing cells taken in the entire body of a flu sufferer whose body was preserved in permafrost because he had been buried in 1918.

Etymology

Despite its title, epidemiological and historic data can't identify the origin of the flu. The source of this "Spanish influenza" title comes out of the pandemic's spread to Spain from France in November 1918. Spain wasn't involved having stayed neutral, and hadn't enforced censorship during wartime. Newspapers were free to report the epidemic's effects, like the grave illness of King Alfonso XIII, and such widely-spread stories generated a false belief. Almost a century after the influenza struck in 1918--1920, the World Health Oganization (WHO) called on scientists, national governments and the press to follow best practices in discovering fresh human infectious diseases to minimize unnecessary adverse consequences on states, economies and individuals. More modern terms with this virus comprise the "1918 flu pandemic," the "1918 influenza pandemic," or variants of them.

Hypotheses Concerning The Origin

British Troops In France

The UK troop hospital and staging camp at Étaples in Virologist John Oxford has speculated France as being in the middle of the flu. His analysis found that with high mortality, which caused symptoms like the flu, the Étaples camp had been struck by the beginning of a disease at 1916. Based on Oxford, a similar outbreak occurred in March 1917 at military barracks at Alders, and military pathologists afterwards realized these premature outbreaks were the exact same disorder as the 1918 influenza. Hospital and the camp were perfect sites for dispersing the virus. The hospital treated 100,000 soldiers, victims of warfare, and chemical attacks. It was home to a piggery, and poultry had been brought in for food supplies in villages. His group and oxford declared that a metric virus, sailed to pigs and harbored in critters, mutated. A report printed in 2016 at the Journal of the Chinese Medical Association discovered signs that the 1918 virus was circulating in the European armies for months and maybe years prior to the 1918 pandemic.

United States

There have been announcements that the outbreak originated in the United States. Historian Alfred W. Crosby said in 2003 that the influenza originated in Kansas, and popular writer John M. Barry explained a January 1918 outbreak in Haskell County, Kansas as the point of origin from his 2004 article. A 2018 analysis of tissue slides and clinical reports directed by evolutionary research scientist Michael Worobec discovered evidence contrary to the disorder arising out of Kansas, as these instances had fewer deaths when compared with the situation in NYC at precisely the exact same period of time. The study failed to find signs; though it wasn't conclusive, the virus had a source. Additionally, the haemagglutinin glycoproteins of the virus imply that it had been around long until 1918 along with another research imply that the reassortment of the H1N1 virus probably occurred in roughly 1915.

China

Among the regions of the world apparently influenced from the 1918 influenza pandemic was China, in which there might have been a relatively mild flu season in 1918 (though this is disputed because of absence of information throughout the Warlord Period of China, visit Around the world). Studies have reported that there were deaths in comparison to other areas of earth. This has caused speculation that the 1918 influenza pandemic originated in China. Rates of influenza mortality in China in 1918 and the flu season might be clarified by the population acquired immunity to the influenza virus. In 1993, the expert for the Pasteur Institute about the 1918 flu, Claude Hannoun, claimed the virus was likely to have come from China. It then mutated in the USA near Boston and from there spread to Brest, France, Europe's battlefields, Europe, and the planet with Allied soldiers and sailors as the main disseminators. In 2014, historian Mark Humphries contended the mobilization of all laborers to operate behind the French and British lines could have been the origin of the pandemic. Humphries, of the Memorial University of Newfoundland in St. John's, based his decisions on recently unearthed records. He discovered evidence was identified by health officials equal to the flu. A report printed in 2016 at the Journal of the Chinese Medical Association found no signs that the 1918 virus had been imported to Europe through Chinese and Southeast Asian soldiers and employees, butinstead found signs of its flow in Europe prior to the pandemic. The 2016 study indicated that the very low flu mortality rate (an estimated 1/1000) found one of the Chinese and Southeast Asian employees in Europe meant the deadly 1918 flu pandemic couldn't have originated from these employees. A 2018 analysis of tissue slides and clinical reports directed by evolutionary research scientist Michael Worobey discovered evidence contrary to the disease being distributed by Chinese employees, noting that employees entered Europe via other avenues, which didn't lead to detectable spread, making them unlikely to have been the original hosts.

Additional

Hannoun considered different hypotheses of source, like Spain, Kansas, and Brest, as potential, but not probable. Political scientist Andrew Price-Smith published information in the archives in Austria, 1917.

Spread

When an infected person sneezes or coughs, million virus particles can disperse to people nearby. Troop movements of World War I and close quarters hastened both transmissions, and likely the pandemic and mutation that were augmented. The lethality of the virus might have increased. Some speculate that the soldiers' immune systems were weakened, in addition to by malnourishment. An element in the occurrence of the flu was raised journey. Modern transport systems made it much easier for sailors, soldiers, and even travelers to spread the illness. The following was refusal and lies by authorities.

The disorder was observed in Haskell County, Kansas, in January 1918, prompting local physician Loring Miner to frighten that the US Public Health Service's educational diary. About 4 March 1918, firm cook Albert Gitchell, from Haskell County, reported ill at Fort Riley, a US military facility that at the time had been training American troops during World War I, making him the first recorded victim of the influenza. In days, guys in the camp had reported ill. About 11 Queens had been conquered by the virus. Everyone was struggling to take steps to counter it but their actions were criticized. In August 1918, a more virulent strain appeared concurrently in Brest, France; at Freetown, Sierra

Leone; and at the U.S., in September, in the Boston Navy Yard and Camp Devens (later renamed Fort Devens), roughly 30 kilometers west of Boston. Other U.S. military websites were shortly affected, as were soldiers being hauled to Europe. By returning soldiers, the influenza carried there.

Mortality

Around The World

The influenza effected about a quarter of the planet's inhabitants. Estimates as to how many infected individuals died vary considerably, but the influenza was not regarded as among the deadliest pandemics. A quote from 1991 claims that the virus killed between 25 and 39 million individuals. A 2005 estimate put the death toll in 50 million (less than 3 percent of the worldwide population), and maybe as large as 100 million (greater than 5 percent). However, a reassessment at 2018 estimated the total to be approximately 17 million, although this was contested. With a world population of 1.8 to 1.9 billion, these estimates correspond between 1 and 6% of the populace. This influenza killed more people than The Black Death, that lasted longer, murdered a proportion of the world's smaller inhabitants. The illness killed in regions of the planet. A few 12-17 million people died roughly 5 percent of the populace, in India. The death toll in India's British-ruled districts was 13.88 million. Arnold (2019) quotes at least 12 million deceased. Estimates for its death toll in China have varied, which reflects the absence of group of health data. The first quote of this Chinese death toll has been created in 1991 by Patterson and Pyle, which estimated China needed a death toll of between 5 and 9 million. But studies as a result of faulty methodology criticized this 1991 analysis, and studies have released estimates of a mortality rate in China. As an example, Iijima in 1998 estimates that the death toll in China to be between 1 and 1.28 million according to information accessible Chinese port towns. Since, Wataru Iijima notes,' Pyle and Patterson within their research 'The 1918 Influenza Pandemic' attempted to gauge the amount of deaths as a whole from the flu in China. They contended between 4.0 and 9.5 million people died in China, yet this total was established purely on the premise that the passing rate there was 1.0--2.25 percent in 1918, since China was a bad nation very similar to Indonesia and India in which the mortality rate was of the purchase. Their analysis wasn't based on any statistical information. The lower estimates of the Chinese death toll derive from the minimal mortality rates, which were discovered in Chinese port towns (by way of instance, Hong Kong) and also on the premise that poor communications prevented the influenza from entering the inside of China. But some modern post and newspaper office reports, in addition to reports from missionary physicians, imply the influenza failed to penetrate the Chinese inside and that flu was awful in certain places in the countryside of China.

23 million people were affected; with at least deaths were reported by 390,000. From the Dutch East Indies (now Indonesia), 1.5 million were supposed to have expired among 30 million individuals. In Tahiti, 13 percent of the people died during a month. In the same way, in just two months, 22 percent of the populace of 38,000 died at Samoa. In New Zealand, the flu killed an estimated 6,400 Pakeha and 2,500 native Maori in fourteen days, together with Māori expiring at eight times the speed of Pakeha.

In Iran, the Mortality was quite high:

•   According to a quote, 8 to 22 percent of the population, or involving 902,400 and 2,431,000 expired.

In the U.S., roughly 28 percent of the Populace of 105 million became infected, and 500,000 to 850,000 expired (0.48 to 0.81 percentage of the populace). Native American tribes were hard hit. There have been deaths among Americans. Alaskan village communities and whole Inuit expired in Alaska. 50,000 expired. In Britain, as many as in France, Alves Back in Brazil, over 400,000. In Ghana, at least 100,000 individuals were killed by the flu epidemic. Tafari Makonnen (the near future Haile Selassie, Emperor of Ethiopia) was among those earliest Ethiopians who contracted flu but lived. Many of the subjects didn't; quotes for deaths from the capital city include even higher or even 5,000 to 10,000. In British Somaliland, 1 official estimated that 7 percent of the population died. This death toll caused from an infection rate of the seriousness of these symptoms and also around 50%, suspected to be brought on by storms. Symptoms in 1918 were uncommon causing flu. 1 contributor wrote, "Among the most notable of these complications was hemorrhage from mucous membranes, particularly from the nose, stomach, and intestine. Bleeding from the ears and petechial hemorrhages in skin also happened". The vast majority of deaths have been a secondary disease, from pneumonia. By inducing hemorrhages and edema in the 15, the virus murdered people.

Patterns Of Fatality

Adults were killed by the pandemic. Back in 1918–1919, 99

percent of pandemic flu deaths from the U.S. happened in people under 65, and almost half of deaths were in young adults 20 to 40 years old. The mortality rate among people under 65 had diminished six-fold but 92 percent of deaths occurred in people. Because the flu is generally deadly to individuals, like infants under age 2 and the immune compromised, this is uncommon. Back in 1918, older adults might have experienced partial protection brought on by exposure to the 1889-1890 influenza pandemic, called the "Russian flu." Based on historian John M. Barry, the most exposed of– "those probably, of the very likely", to perish -- were pregnant ladies. He reported in thirteen researches of women in the pandemic, the death rate ranged from 23 to 71 percent. Of those pregnant women who lived childbirth, over one-quarter (26 percent) dropped the kid. The other oddity was that the epidemic was prevalent at the summer and fall (from the Northern Hemisphere); flu is generally worse in the winter. Contemporary research has proven that the virus to be especially deadly because it activates a cytokine storm (overreaction of the body's immune system), which ravages the more powerful immune system of young adults. The virus was retrieved by 1 set of investigators in the bodies of creatures that were transfected and victims with it. The creatures suffered progressive respiratory failure and passing. Whereas the poorer reactions of adults and kids resulted in deaths, the immune reactions of adults have been postulated to have shattered the entire body. By consolidation, mortality has been mostly in scenarios. Cases comprised neural involvement that led sometimes to mental disorders, and bacterial infections. Some deaths were the result of malnourishment. A research conducted employed a mechanistic modeling approach to examine the 3 waves of the 1918 flu pandemic. They analyzed the elements that underlie variability in their significance and patterns to patterns of morbidity and mortality. Their analysis indicates that the explanation is provided by variations in transmission speed, and also the variation is inside plausible values. Another analysis by The et al. (2013) employed a simple epidemic model comprising three variables to infer the reason for the 3 waves of the 1918 flu pandemic. These variables were closure and college opening, temperature changes during the outbreak, and individual modifications in response to this outbreak. The consequences were shown by behavioral reactions, although their modeling results demonstrated that all three variables are significant. A 2020 analysis found that US towns, which implemented extensive and early non-medical measures (quarantine etc.) endured no further adverse financial consequences because of implementing those steps, compared to cities that implemented steps late or in any way.

Deadly Second Tide

The wave of the 1918 pandemic was more deadly compared to first. The wave had resembled flu epidemics; people most in danger were older and the ill, whereas fitter people recovered. From August, once the second wave started in Sierra Leone France and the USA, the virus had mutated into a form. October 1918 was the month with the maximum fatality rate of the pandemic in its entirety. This seriousness was credited to the conditions of the First World War. In life, a strain is favored by natural selection. From the trench's selection was reversed. Where they had been soldiers with a strain remained, while the ill were sent to area hospitals to trains, dispersing the more deadly virus. The second wave started, and the entire world was spread across by the influenza. Thus, during modern pandemics, health officials listen once the virus reaches areas with societal upheaval (searching for deadlier strains of this virus). The simple fact that the majority of people who recovered from ailments that were first-wave had become immune revealed that it has to have been the strain of influenza. This was dramatically exemplified in Copenhagen, which escaped using a joint mortality rate of just 0.29percent (0.02 percent in the initial wave and 0.27 percent in the next wave) due to vulnerability to the less-lethal first tide. For the remaining portion of the populace, the next wave was much more mortal; the individuals that were most exposed were those such as the soldiers in the trenches -- adults that were fit and youthful.

Devastated Communities

Mass graves were dug by steam shovel and bodies buried without coffins in many areas. Pacific island lands were hit hard. The pandemic reached them from New Zealand, which had been slow to execute measures to stop from leaving its vents, boats, like the SS Talune, taking the flu. By New Zealand, the influenza attained Tonga (murdering 8 percent of the populace), Nauru (16 percent), and Fiji (5 percent, 9,000 individuals). Worst was Western Samoa German Samoa that was inhabited by New Zealand in 1914. 90 percent of the population was infected; 22 percent of women 30 percent of men, and 10 percent of kids died. By comparison, the flu was prevented by Governor John Martin Poyer by means of a blockade from reaching American Samoa. The disease spread quickest through the social

194

groups among the peoples, due to the habit of collecting heritage from chiefs in their deathbed's community elders were infected through this procedure. In New Zealand, 8,573 deaths have been attributed to the 1918 pandemic flu, leading to an entire population fatality rate of 0.7 percent. Māori were 8 to 10 times less likely to die as Pakeha, due to the comparative poverty, more crowded home, rural inhabitants and lesser resistance to illness. In 1918, the influenza accounted for 10 percent of the deaths in Ireland.

Less-Affected Places

China might have undergone a mild flu season in 1918 in comparison to other regions of the planet. There was no group of health data in the nation at the moment, and a few reports out of its inside indicate that mortality rates from flu were greater in at least a few places in China. At the minimum, there's minimal proof that the influenza affected China as a whole in contrast to other nations on earth. Though records from the inside of China are missing, there was information listed in, like Harbin, Canton, Peking, Hong Kong and Shanghai. The Chinese Maritime Customs Service that has been staffed by foreigners, like the British, French, and other colonial officials in China gathered this information. As a complete, low mortality rates are shown by true data from the port towns of China in comparison to other towns in Asia. For instance, the British government at Hong Kong and Canton reported a mortality rate from flu at a speed of 0.25 and 0.32 percent, considerably lower than the reported mortality rate of different cities in Asia, for example Calcutta or Bombay, at which flu was a lot more catastrophic. From Shanghai's city -- that had a population of more than 2 million that there were only 266 deaths from flu among the people in 1918. If extrapolated in the extensive data listed from Chinese towns, the proposed mortality rate from flu in China as a whole in 1918 was probably lower than 1 percent -- considerably lower than the world average (that was approximately 3--5 percent). By comparison, Japan and Taiwan had reported a mortality rate from flu around 0.45% and 0.69% respectively, greater than the mortality rate accumulated from statistics in Chinese port cities, including Hong Kong (0.25 percent), Canton (0.32 percent), and Shanghai. Back in Japan, 257,363 deaths have been attributed to the flu by July 1919, providing an estimated 0.4 percent mortality rate, which was considerably lower than almost all other Asian nations for which data are readily available. When the pandemic struck, the authorities restricted sea traveling to and from.

In American Samoa, the Pacific and the colony of New Caledonia succeeded in preventing a single death through quarantines. Almost 12,000 expired. From the conclusion of the island of Marajó, the pandemic in Brazil's Amazon River Delta hadn't reported an outbreak. No deaths were reported by Saint Helena. The passing although the epidemiologists that toll in Russia was estimated at 450,000. If it is right, Russia lost percent of its inhabitants -- the lowest mortality in Asia. This is considered by another study. The infrastructure of life had broken down Death toll was closer to 2 percent, or 2.7 million people.

Aspirin Poisoning

In 2009, a paper printed in the journal Clinical Infectious Karen Starko suggested that aspirin poisoning contributed to the deaths. She based that on the reported symptoms of people dying from the flu, as mentioned from the post mortem reports still accessible, as well as the timing of this large "departure spike" in October 1918. This happened shortly after the Surgeon General of the U.S. Army, along with the Journal of the American Medical Association, both advocated quite massive doses of 2 to 31 grams of aspirin daily as part of therapy. These amounts created hyperventilation in lung edema in 3 percent of patients, in addition to 33 percent of patients. Starko additionally notes that lots of premature deaths demonstrated "moist," occasionally hemorrhagic lungs, whereas late deaths revealed bacterial pneumonia. She indicates that the tide of aspirin poisonings was the result of a "perfect storm" of events: Bayer's patent on aspirin died, so many companies rushed in to earn a gain and significantly increased the source; this collaborated with the Spanish influenza; and the indications of aspirin poisoning weren't known at the moment. For example, for its high mortality rate, this theory was contested in a letter to the journal printed in April 2010 by Andrew Noymer and Daisy Carreon of the University of California, Irvine, and Niall Johnson of the Australian Commission on Safety and Quality in Healthcare. They contested the applicability of this aspirin concept, given that the high mortality rate in which there was no or little access to aspirin in the moment, in contrast to the death rate in areas. They reasoned that "the salicylate aspirin poisoning theory was hard to maintain as the most important explanation for the unusual virulence of the 1918-1919 flu pandemic." In reaction, Starko stated there was scientific evidence of aspirin usage in India and contended that if aspirin over-prescription hadn't contributed to the elevated Indian mortality rate, it might still happen to be a factor for elevated rates in locations where other exacerbating factors found in India played a function.

End Of The Pandemic

Following the deadly wave struck instances that are fresh, in 1918 dropped from the wave. By way of instance, 4,597 people died in the week ending 16 October, but from town, the flu had vanished by 11 November. One explanation for the rapid decrease from the lethality of this disease is that physicians became effective in prevention and therapy of their pneumonia that developed following the sufferers that contracted the virus. Some cases that are mortal did last into March 1919. Another theory maintains that the 1918 virus mutated into a strain. This is a frequent phenomenon with flu viruses: there's a trend for pathogenic viruses to be less deadly with time, as the hosts of dangerous breeds have a tendency to expire (see also "Deadly Second Wave", above).

Long-Term Consequences

That was discovered by a 2006 research from the Journal of Political Economy "cohorts in utero" during the pandemic demonstrated reduced educational attainment, improved degrees of physical handicap, lower earnings, lower socioeconomic status, and greater transfer payments received in comparison to other birth cohorts. A 2018 research discovered that the pandemic decreased educational attainment in populations. The flu was connected from the 1920s to the epidemic of encephalitis lethargica.

• Chapter - 3 What's Spanish Flu?

This influenza is also called the 1918 influenza pandemic, or the deadly flu. Lasting from January 1918 500 million people -- roughly a third of the planet's population – were infected by it. The death toll was estimated to have been everywhere from as large as 100 million, and 17 million to 50 million, which makes it among the deadliest pandemics in history. World War I censored diminished reports of mortality and illness in the USA, the UK, France, and Germany to preserve sanity. Newspapers were free to report the epidemic's effects in neutral Spain, like the grave illness of King Alfonso XIII, and such stories generated a false belief of Spain as particularly hard hit. This gave rise. Ancient and epidemiological data are insufficient to identify with certainty that the pandemics geographical source, with varying perspectives regarding its place. Most flu outbreaks kill the very young and the very old, using a greater survival rate for all those in between, but the Spanish influenza pandemic led to a greater than expected mortality rate for adults. Researchers provide several explanations for its high mortality rate of the 1918 flu pandemic. Some investigations have demonstrated the virus to be especially deadly because it activates a cytokine storm, which ravages the more powerful immune system of young adults. By comparison, a 2007 analysis of health care journals in the length of the pandemic discovered that the viral disease was not any more competitive than previous flu strains. Rather, hygiene, overcrowded spas and hospitals, and malnourishment encouraged infection. This infection was deadly to all victims. The Spanish influenza was the first of 2 pandemics caused by the flu virus; the next was that influenza in 2009.

What's The Flu?

Influenza, or flu, is a virus that attacks the respiratory system. The influenza virus is extremely infectious: If an infected person coughs, sneezes or talks, respiratory droplets are created and transmitted to the atmosphere, and may be inhaled by anyone near. Furthermore, someone who rolls something with the entire virus onto it and then touches their mouth, nose, or eyes may get infected. Flu outbreaks occur annually and change in severity, depending in part on which sort of virus is spreading. (Flu viruses can quickly mutate.)

Spanish Influenza: The Virus That Changed The World

A disorder started to sweep a deadly virus that infected a third of the planet's inhabitants and left upwards of 50 million dead. Laura Spinney investigated the devastating effect of the Spanish influenza pandemic and how it contrasted the Coronavirus disaster on 28 September 1918. A Spanish paper gave its viewers a brief lesson on flu. "The representative responsible for this disease, it is your Pfeiffer's bacillus, which is very tiny and observable only by way of a microscope." The explanation was because the entire world was in the grasp of their very barbarous influenza pandemic on record -- but it was wrong: influenza is caused by a virus. The concept that influenza was caused by a bacillus or Illness was approved by the most distinguished scientists of their day, who'd find themselves almost completely helpless in the face of the scourge.

Just How Many People Died From The Spanish Flu?

Spanish influenza was among the deadliest disasters in history. It lasted for 2 decades -- between the earliest documented instance in March 1918 and the past in March 1920, an estimated 50 million people died, although some experts indicate that the total could have been double. Even the 'Spanish flu' murdered during the First World War, maybe more than the Second World War.

How Can Spanish Influenza Compare To Coronavirus?Laura Spinney told me "You may have observed a figure floating about of a case fatality rate of 3.4 percent, which describes the ratio of individuals who capture the COVID-19 disease who go to die of it. The amount that is frequently quoted for its Spanish Flu, as an instance, the case fatality rate is 2.5percent but it is a very, very, very controversial figure since the amounts are so obscure. I mean we believe that probably 50 million people died but there wasn't any kind of reliable test in the time so that we cannot be convinced about that which only cries all of the numbers out." So, it is really tough to create the historic comparisons, even in the event that you've got accurate data today, which we do not. Therefore, on either side of the equation, even if you prefer, it is a moving target. "We'd obviously love to get a vaccine from COVID-19 today but we do not and we might need to wait a year to 18 months because of that. They'd have no vaccine whatsoever in 1918. Or rather they did create molds but they were unworthy, pretty much, as they were basically pathogens against bacteria in the respiratory tract whereas, as we understand, influenza is a viral illness. So,

regarding this, we're advanced compared to 1918. But we do not have that vaccine. We have anti-inflammatory medication for treating the ill and we have antibiotics that will be useful for treating the bacterial ailments that might lead to pneumonia sometimes, as they did in 1918, interestingly."

The pandemic struck in a vital juncture of comprehension of illness that is infectious. Well into the 19th century, epidemics were considered acts of God -- a belief that dated back into the Middle Ages. Originally, although compounds were observed in the 17th century, they were not connected with disorders. In the 1850s, the French biologist Louis Pasteur made the link between disorder and micro-organisms, and by a couple of microbiologist Robert Koch furthered notions of illness. 'Germ concept' was disseminated far and wide, replacing thoughts that were fatalistic. The 20th century, together with improvements in sanitation and hygiene, had made considerable inroads from the so-called 'audience' ailments that affected human communities, particularly those inhabiting the fantastic cities which had mushroomed in the aftermath of the industrial revolution. Through the 19th century many urbanites were dropped to diseases -- cholera, tuberculosis, and typhus, to mention three -- which cities had a continuous influx of peasants in the countryside to keep their numbers up. At last they had become self-explanatory.

Where Did The Spanish Flu Originate? Some

theories suggest it did not begin in Spain. We do not understand where it began, but we know it did not begin in Spain. The Spanish were, to a degree, stigmatized with this. Even though the trenches of the First World War are still a contender, there's also no means of being sure where Spanish

Flu originated. The soldiers' immune system changed. It's believed before spreading at an alarming speed to Europe, the cases were the pandemic was known as 'Spanish Flu.' Censorship exaggerated the effects of the virus in Spain. While Britain, France, Germany, and the USA censored and limited early reports, newspapers in Spain -- as a neutral nation -- were liberated to communicate all of the dreadful details of this pandemic.

From 1918, faith in mathematics was low, and large scientists had adopted a swagger. Twenty years before, this had motivated the Irish playwright George Bernard Shaw to compose the physician's Dilemma, where an eminent physician, Sir Colenso Ridgeon -- a personality according to Sir Almroth Wright, who developed the typhoid vaccine -- plays god with his patients' destinies. Shaw was warning physicians against hubris; however, it required an epidemic of another 'audience' disorder -- flu -- to bring them home they understood. When scientists believed about 'germs' from the 20th century, they thought about germs. The virus was a novel theory; its capacity had infected tobacco plants and discovered the virus, found in 1892. Unlike germs, it had been too little to be viewed through an optical microscope. Without having really observed viruses, scientists mimicked their character. They had been veiled in mystery, and no one guessed that they might be the reason for the flu. Throughout the influenza pandemic -- the so-called 'Russian' flu, which started in 1889 -- a pupil of Koch's called Richard Pfeiffer promised to have identified. Pfeiffer's bacillus, as it had been known, can cause illness and does exist -- but it doesn't cause flu. During the 1918 pandemic, pathologists who cultivated bacterial colonies in the lung tissue of influenza victims discovered Pfeiffer's bacillus in certain, but not all of the civilizations, which puzzled them. To add to physicians' puzzlement, vaccines generated from the bacillus of Pfeiffer appeared to gain some patients. Actually, these experiments were successful against secondary bacterial diseases that caused pneumonia -- that the greatest cause of death in most instances -- but scientists did not understand that at the moment. They'd realize that it was a mistake.

Flu Season

In the USA, "flu season" normally runs from late Fall into spring. In a normal year, over 200,000 Americans are hospitalized for flu-related complications, and within the last 3 decades, there were several 3,000 to 49,000 flu-related U.S. deaths annually, according to the Centers for Disease Control and Prevention. Young kids, individuals over age 65, pregnant women, and individuals with particular medical conditions, like diabetes, asthma, or cardiovascular disease, face a greater chance of flu-related complications, such as pneumonia, sinus, ear infections and hepatitis. Influenza pandemic, like the one in 1918, happens when a particularly virulent new flu strain for which there is little if any immunity arises and spreads rapidly from person to person around the world.

Spanish Flu Symptoms

The initial wave of the 1918 pandemic happened in the spring and was mild. The ill, which underwent such common influenza symptoms like chills, fatigue, and fever, normally recovered after a few days, and also the number of reported deaths was reduced. The second wave of flu appeared in the autumn of that year with a vengeance. Victims died within days or hours of symptoms. By a couple of years, the average life expectancy in America dropped 1918, in 1 year.

What Led To The Spanish Flu?

It is unknown exactly where the specific breed of Flu that caused the pandemic originated. Nonetheless, the 1918 influenza was first detected in Europe, America, and regions of Asia before spreading to nearly every other portion of the world in a matter of weeks. Regardless of the fact that the 1918 influenza was not isolated to a location, it became famous around the world since Spanish influenza, Spain was struck hard by the illness and wasn't subject to the malevolent news blackouts that affected other European nations. (Spain's king, Alfonso XIII, allegedly contracted the flu) 1 odd aspect of the 1918 influenza was that it struck many formerly healthy, young individuals – a band generally resistant to this form of infectious disease – including lots of World War I servicemen. In reality, many more U.S. soldiers died from the 1918 influenza than were killed in the conflict during the war. Forty percent of the U.S. Navy was struck with the flu, while 36% of the Army became sick. Soldiers moving around the planet in crowded trains and ships helped to disperse the killer virus. Additional estimates run as large as 3% of the planet's inhabitants. The death toll attributed to the influenza is estimated at 20 million to 50 million sufferers globally. The numbers are not possible to understand because of a deficiency of health. What is known is that places were resistant to the 1918 influenza – to people of communities that were remote, victims ranged from residents of cities in America. Even President Woodrow Wilson allegedly contracted influenza in early 1919 while negotiating the Treaty of Versailles, which ended World War I.

Why Was The Spanish Flu Called Spanish?

The Spanish Flu didn't arise in Spain. Spain was a state with a press that covered the outbreak in Madrid in May from the beginning. Meanwhile, the Central Powers, as well as Allied nations, had censors who covered news of this influenza up to keep morale high. Since Spanish information resources were not the only ones reporting on influenza, many considered it originated there (the Spanish, meanwhile, considered the virus originated out of France and called it the "French Flu.")

Where Did The Spanish Flu Come From?

Scientists do not know for certain where the Flu originated. Concepts point to France, China, Britain, and also the USA, in which the earliest instance was reported on March 11, 1918, in Camp Funston at Fort Riley, Kansas. Some consider soldiers that were infected had spread the illness throughout the nation to army camps. In March 1918, the subsequent month soldiers led across the Atlantic and have been followed closely by 118,000 more.

First Instances Reported From The Deadly Spanish Influenza Pandemic

Before breakfast on the afternoon of March 4, Albert Mitchell of the U.S. Army reports on the hospital in Fort Riley, Kansas, whining of those cold-like symptoms of sore throat, pain, and fever. By comparison, over 100 of his fellow soldiers had reported symptoms that were similar, signaling what are thought to be the initial cases from the flu pandemic of 1918. Influenza would kill an estimated 20 million to 50 million people and 675,000 Americans across the world, proving to be a much more deadly force than the First World War. The outbreak of this disease has been accompanied by outbreaks in prisons and military camps in a variety of areas of the nation. The disease shortly traveled to Europe together with the American soldiers going to help the Allies in the battlefields of France (Back in March 1918 alone, 84,000 American soldiers led across the Atlantic; yet another 118,000 followed them another month). Influenza revealed no signs of abating when it came on another continent: 31,000 cases were reported in Great Britain in June. The disorder was soon dubbed Spanish influenza as a result of a shockingly higher number of deaths in Spain (some 8 million, it had been reported) following the first outbreak there in May 1918. No mercy was shown by influenza on each side of the trenches for combatants. The initial wave of the outbreak hit against German forces, in which they waged a closing offensive which could establish the results of the war. It had a substantial impact on the morale of their troops as the flu deepened losses, along with bad provisions depressing the spirits of guys in the III Infantry Division. The flu spread past the boundaries of Western Europe. The close of the summer had cases reported in Russia, North Africa, and India; New Zealand, Japan, the Philippines as well as China would fall victim. The Great War ended on November 11, but flu continued to wreak global havoc, flaring again in the U.S. within a more vicious wave together with the return of soldiers against the war and finally infecting an estimated 28 percent of the nation's population before it eventually petered out.

Fighting The Spanish Flu

Scientists and doctors were unsure after the 1918 flu strike what caused it or how to take care of it. There were drugs which treated the flu but no vaccines or antivirals. (The very first accredited flu vaccine emerged in America in the 1940s. By the next decade, vaccine makers could routinely create vaccines that would help restrain and protect against potential pandemics). Complicating matters was the fact that World War I had abandoned a lack of doctors and other health workers to portions of America. And of that available medical personnel from the U.S., many came back with the flu themselves. Hospitals in certain areas were bombarded with influenza patients who other buildings, private houses, and schools needed to be converted to hospitals, a few of which were staffed with students. Officials in certain areas imposed quarantines such as churches, schools, and theaters. People were advised also to remain inside and also to avoid shaking hands, libraries placed a block on regulations and financing books. According to the New York Times, throughout the ordeal, Boy Scouts in New York approached people they had seen spitting on the road and gave them cards which read: "You're in violation of this Sanitary Code."

Aspirin Poisoning And The Flu

Without treatment for the flu physicians, they believed it would relieve symptoms. For example: aspirin, which was trademarked by Bayer in 1899 – a patent which died in 1917, meaning fresh firms could create the medication during the Spanish Flu outbreak. Prior to the spike in deaths attributed to the Spanish Flu in 1918, the U.S. Surgeon General, Navy and also the Journal of the American Medical Association had recommended the use of aspirin. Medical professionals counseled patients to take around 30g every day. (For comparison's sake, the health consensus now is that doses over 4g is dangerous). Indicators of aspirin poisoning include the buildup of fluid in the lungs, or hyperventilation, and edema, and it believed that a number hastened or of those October deaths were caused by aspirin poisoning.

The Flu Takes Heavy Toll On Society

Influenza took countless lives; creating widows and orphans. Funeral parlors were filled with bodies as they began piling up. People needed to dig graves for their very own Relatives. The influenza was injurious to the market. From the United States, because many workers stated they were forced to shut down sick. Basic services like trash collection and mail delivery were hindered due to employees. There were farm employees to harvest plants. Even local and state health departments shut down for company, hampering attempts to supply and to chronicle the spread of the 1918 influenza People about it with responses.

The Way U.S. Cities Try To Stop The 1918 Flu Pandemic

A catastrophic tide of the Spanish Flu struck American beaches in the summer of 1918 and spread to various cities. With no vaccine or treatment program, it dropped to officials and mayors to improvise plans to protect the citizens. With pressure to appear patriotic at wartime and with a censored media downplaying the disease's spread, many made tragic decisions. The answer to Philadelphia was too little, too late. Dr. Wilmer Krusen, manager of Public Health and Charities for the town, insisted mounting deaths weren't the "Spanish flu," but instead the only influenza. The town moved with a

Liberty Loan parade spreading the illness. More than 1,000 Philadelphians were lifeless. Only then did the city close saloons and theaters. From March 1919, their own lives had been lost by over 15,000 citizens of Philadelphia. St. Louis, Missouri, was distinct: Schools and film theaters closed and public parties were prohibited. As a result, the peak mortality rate in St. Louis was only one-eighth of Philadelphia's passing rate during the peak of the outbreak. Citizens at San Francisco were fined $5 when they had been caught with no masks and charged with disturbing the peace.

Spanish Flu Pandemic Ends

From the summer of 1919, the influenza pandemic came to an end; those who were infected either acquired resistance or expired. Nearly 90 decades after, in 2008, researchers announced they had found exactly what made the 1918 flu so fatal: A bunch of 3 genes allowed the virus to weaken a sufferer's bronchial tubes and lungs and clear the way for bacterial pneumonia. Too lethal, there were other flu pandemics since 1918. An influenza pandemic from 1957 to 1958 killed around two million people globally, such as some 70,000 people in America, along with also a pandemic from 1968 to 1969 killed approximately 1 million individuals, including some 34,000 Americans. Over 12,000 Americans expired during the H1N1 (or "swine flu") pandemic, which happened from 2009 to 2010. The novel coronavirus outbreak of 2020 is spreading around the globe as nations race to locate a remedy for COVID 19 and taxpayers refuge set up in an effort to prevent spreading the illness, which can be very deadly because most carriers are asymptomatic for times before recognizing they're infected. Every one of those modern-day pandemics brings renewed attention in and focus on the Spanish Flu, or "forgotten pandemic," so-named since its spread had been overshadowed by the deadliness of both WWI and coated by information blackouts and inadequate record-keeping.

Chapter - 4 Why Can It Be Known As 'Spanish Flu'?

Influenza had obtained its name as it had been thought to have originated from Bukhara in Uzbekistan (at the time, part of the Russian empire). The pandemic, which broke out almost 30 decades after will always be called the 'Spanish flu', although it did not begin in Spain. It washed across the entire world in three waves that, at the northern hemisphere, corresponded to some gentle wave in the spring of 1918, a deadly wave the subsequent fall, and reprisal from the first months of 1919, which was intermediate in virulence between both. The cases were listed at Camp Funston. Within six weeks that the illness had reached the trenches of the western front in France, however, it was only in May that influenza broke out in Spain. Contrary to the USA and France, Spain was neutral in the war; therefore it did not censor its own press. The first Spanish instances were reported in the papers, also since King Alfonso XIII, the prime minister, and many members of this cabinet were one of those early cases; the nation's plight was highly observable. People around the world thought that the disorder had rippled from Madrid -- a misconception encouraged by propagandists in these belligerent countries that knew they had contracted it before Spain. In the interest of maintaining morale high within their populations, they were pleased to change the blame. The title stuck. Understandably, Spaniards smarted at this calumny: they understood that they weren't accountable, and imagined the French of getting sent influenza throughout the boundary, but they could not be convinced. They throw around for another tag, also found inspiration in an operetta performed in the capital Zarzuela Theatre -- a hugely popular reworking of the myth of Don Juan, with a catchy song called 'The Soldier of Naples'. The tricky disease became famous in Spain as the 'Naples Soldier.' Although the Spanish flu did not begin in Spain that nation did suffer very badly with it. From the early 20th century, influenza was regarded as a democratic disorder -- nobody was immune against it but, in the thick of this pandemic, it had been noticed that the disease struck. It 'favored' particular age classes: the very young and the older, but also a center cohort aged 20 to 40. It favored men to women, with the exclusion of pregnant ladies, who have been at especially large risk. This age and gender-related patterns have been replicated all around the planet, however, the virulence with influenza struck varied from place to place. Inhabitants of particular parts of Asia have been a shocking 30 times more likely to die from the flu than people in areas of Europe. Generally, Asia and Africa suffered maximum death rates, together with the cheapest found in Europe, North America, and Australia. However, there was great variation in continents, also. African countries south of the Sahara experienced death speeds two or even three times greater than those north of the desert, whereas Spain listed among the maximum passing rates in Europe -- double that in Britain, three times that in Denmark. The unevenness did not stop there. Generally, cities endured worse than rural places, but a few cities endured worse than many others, and there was also variation in towns. Newly arrived immigrants tended to die more frequently than older, better-established groups, for example. In the countryside, one village might be decimated while another, apparently similar in every way, got away with a light dose.

What Kinds Of People Caught The Spanish Flu?

Influenza appeared to attack with an element of randomness and cruelty. Since adults in their prime died in droves, unlucky communities imploded. Kids were orphaned, older parents made to fend for them. Individuals were at a loss to explain this clear lottery, and it left them profoundly disturbed. Trying to clarify the feeling that it inspired in him, a French physician in the town of Lyons wrote that it had been rather unlike the "gut pangs" he'd experienced while serving at the front. This has been "a more deep pressure, the feeling of some indefinable terror which had taken hold of the people of the city." It was only afterward when epidemiologists zeroed in on the amounts that patterns started to emerge, and the initial elements of justification were set forward. A number of the variability may be explained by inequalities of wealth and caste -- and, to the extent, it represented these variables: skin color, poor diet, crowded living conditions, and limited access to healthcare weakened the constitution, which makes the poor, immigrants, and cultural minorities more prone to disease. As French historian Patrick Zylberman said: "The virus may have behaved 'democratically,' but the culture it assaulted was hardly egalitarian."

Any other underlying disorder made someone more vulnerable to the Spanish flu, whereas previous exposure to influenza itself modulates the seriousness of a situation. Remote communities without much historic experience of this illness suffered badly, as did cities that were bypassed by the first wave of the pandemic because they were not immunologically 'primed' to the second. As an instance, Rio de Janeiro – the capital of Brazil at the time – received only one wave of flu in October 1918, and experienced a death rate two or three times higher than that recorded in American cities to the north that had received both the spring and autumn waves. And Bristol Bay in Alaska was spared before early 1919, but if the virus eventually gained a foothold it decreased the bay Eskimo inhabitants by 40 percent. Public health efforts made a difference, in spite of the fact that medics didn't know the reason for the disease. Since time immemorial, if contagion is a danger individuals have practiced 'social distancing' -- knowing unconsciously that steering clear of contaminated people increases the prospect of staying healthy. Back in 1918, social distancing took the kind of quarantine zones, isolation wards, and prohibitions on mass parties; in which they had been correctly enforced, these steps slowed the spread. Australia maintained out the autumn wave completely by implementing a successful quarantine in its ports. Exceptions demonstrated the rule. Back in 1918, Persia was a collapsed country after decades of being used as a pawn in the 'Great Game' -- that the battle between the British and the Russians for control of this huge region between the Arabian and Caspian Seas. Its government was weak and almost broke, and it lacked a coherent sanitary infrastructure. Therefore, whenever the flu faded from the northeastern holy city of Mashhad in August 1918, no social distancing measures were enforced. In a fortnight every house and place of business from Mashhad had been infected, and also two-thirds of this city's inhabitants fell ill that autumn. With no limitations on

215

motion, influenza spread thickly with pilgrims, soldiers, and retailers to the four corners of the nation. From now Persia was free of influenza, it had dropped between 8% and 22 percent of its own population (that doubt representing the fact that, in a state in crisis, collecting statistics was barely a priority). Even 8 percent equates to the mortality rate in Ireland.

Where disparities in rates of illness and death were perceived, people's explanations reflected contemporary understanding – or, rather, misunderstanding – of infectious disease. When Charles Darwin laid out his theory of evolution by natural selection in *On the Origin of Species* (1859), he had not intended his ideas to be applied to human societies, but others of his time did just that, creating the 'science' of eugenics. Eugenicists believed that mankind included 'races' and from 1918 their thinking was mainstream. Some eugenicists noticed that sectors of society suffered against influenza, which they credited to some inferiority. They'd incorporated germ theory in their world perspective: when the poor and the working classes were prone to disease, concluded the eugenicists, they only had themselves to blame, since Pasteur had instructed that disease was preventable.

Indian Anxieties

The consequences of the line of thinking are exemplified in India. That land's British colonizers had long taken the view that India was inherently unhygienic, and so had invested little in indigenous healthcare. As many as 18 million Indians died in the pandemic -- that the reduction in numbers of any nation on the planet. However, there was a backlash. Resentment was fueled by the British reply to the spread of influenza. Tensions came to a head with the passage in 1919. This triggered calm protests, and on 13 April British troops fired into an unarmed crowd in Amritsar, murdering countless Indian individuals -- a massacre that galvanized the liberty movement. Uprisings were prompted by influenza elsewhere. The fall of 1918 saw a tide of workers' strikes and protests around the world. Disgruntlement was smoldering since prior to the Russian revolutions of 1917, but influenza fanned the flames by exacerbating what was a dire source situation, also by highlighting inequality. Even well-ordered Switzerland narrowly prevented a civil war in November 1918 following leftwing groups attributed to a large number of influenza deaths from the military on the authorities and army control. There were regions of the planet where individuals hadn't heard of Darwin or germ theory, and in which the people turned into explanations that are more tried-and-tested. From the rural interior of China, as an instance, a lot of individuals still thought that illness had been sent by dragons and demons; they paraded amounts of dinosaurs through the roads in the hope of appeasing the irate spirits. A missionary physician explained going from house to house in Shanxi province in early 1919, and locating scissors put indoors "to ward off demons or perchance to cut them in 2". In the west that was modernized, individuals vacillated death often seemed to strike without rhyme or reason. Many still remembered a more mystical, pre-Darwinian era, and four years of war had worn down psychological defenses. Seeing how their men of science were to assist them, most people came to think that the stunt was an act of god retribution because of their sins. In Zamora -- exactly the exact same Spanish town whose paper said with such confidence the representative of disorder had been Pfeiffer's bacillus -- that the bishop defied the health authorities' ban on mass parties and ordered people to the dinosaurs to placate "God's legitimate anger." This town then recorded among the maximum death tolls from influenza in Spain -- a simple fact of which its inhabitants were conscious, even though they do not appear to have held it from their own bishop. They gave him a trophy in recognition of his attempts to end his or her suffering. This illustrates gulfs were represented by answers to influenza. The 1918 pandemic struck a planet, which was completely unprepared for this, dealing a body blow to scientific hubris, and destabilizing political and social orders for decades ahead.

Chapter - 5 Kinds Of Influenza Viruses

There are four kinds of influenza viruses: A, B, C, and D. Human influenza A, and B viruses cause seasonal epidemics of illness (called the flu season) nearly every winter in the USA. Influenza A virus is the sole flu virus known to induce flu pandemics, i.e., worldwide epidemics of influenza disease. A pandemic can happen when a new, distinct influenza virus emerges, which both infects individuals and has the capacity to spread efficiently between individuals. Influenza type C cause illness and aren't believed to trigger influenza epidemics. Cattle affect aren't known to infect or cause illness in humans. Flu viruses are divided into subtypes based on two proteins on the surface of the virus: hemagglutinin (H) and neuraminidase (N). There are 18 distinct hemagglutinin subtypes and 11 distinct neuraminidase subtypes (H1 via H18 and N1 via N11, respectively). Just 131 subtypes have been discovered in character when there are 198 influenzas A subtype mixes. Present-day subtypes of flu A viruses which routinely circulate in people contain A (H1N1) and A (H3N2). Influenza A subtypes could be further broken down into distinct genetic "clades" and "sub-clades." Watch the "Influenza Viruses" picture below to get a visual depiction of those classifications.

Human Seasonal Influenza Viruses

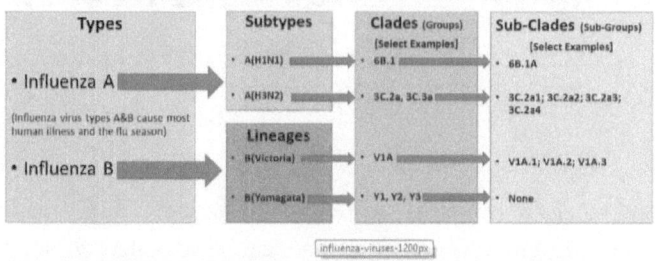

This graphic shows the two types of influenza viruses (A,B) that cause most human illness and that are responsible for the flu season each year. Influenza A viruses are further classified into subtypes, while influenza B viruses are further classified into two lineages: B/Yamagata and B/Victoria. Both influenza A and B viruses can be further classified into specific clades and sub-clades (which are sometimes called groups and sub-groups).

Clades and sub-clades could be rather called "classes" and "sub-groups," respectively. An influenza clade or band is a further subdivision of influenza viruses (past subtypes or lineages) dependent on the similarity of the HA receptor sequences. (Watch the Genome Sequencing and Genetic Characterization page for more info). Clades and subclades are revealed on phylogenetic trees as forms of viruses that normally have comparable genetic changes (i.e., nucleotide or amino acid changes) and also have one common ancestor represented as a node in the tree (see Figure 1). Dividing viruses to clades and subclades enables flu specialists to monitor the ratio of viruses from various clades inflow. Be aware that clades and sub-clades which are genetically distinct from others aren't necessarily antigenically distinct (i.e. viruses out of a particular clade or sub-clade might not have changes that affect host resistance compared with other clades or sub-clades). Currently circulating influenza A(H1N1) viruses are about the pandemic 2009 H1N1 virus, which arose in the spring of 2009 and caused an influenza pandemic (CDC 2009 H1N1 Flu site). This virus clinically referred to as the "A (H1N1) pdm09 virus," and more commonly called "2009 H1N1," has continued to float since then. All these H1N1 viruses have experienced relatively small genetic modifications and modifications to their antigenic properties (i.e., the properties of this virus that influence resistance) as time passes. Of all of the flu viruses which habitually circulate and cause illness in people, influenza A (H3N2) viruses have a tendency to change more quickly, both genetically and antigenically. Influenza A (H3N2) viruses have shaped many different, genetically distinct clades lately, which continue to co-circulate. Influenza B viruses aren't divided into subtypes, but rather are categorized into two lineages: B/Yamagata and B/Victoria. Influenza B viruses may be classified into sub-clades and clades. Influenza B viruses normally change more gradually when it comes to their genetic and antigenic properties compared to influenza A viruses, particularly influenza A(H3N2) viruses. Influenza surveillance data in the last years reveals the co-circulation of influenza B viruses from the lineages from the USA and across the world. The proportion of influenza B viruses that circulate may vary by location.

Influenza Vaccine Viruses

One influenza A (H1N1), one influenza A (H3N2), and one or 2 Influenza B viruses (depending upon the vaccine) are contained in every year's flu vaccines. Obtaining a flu vaccine may protect against influenza viruses, which are similar to the viruses used to make disease. Info concerning the vaccine of this season is located at preventing Seasonal Flu with Vaccination. Influenza vaccines don't protect against flu D or C viruses. Additionally, influenza vaccines won't protect against disease and illness due to other viruses, which also may lead to influenza-like symptoms. There are a number of different viruses besides flu that may lead to influenza-like illness (ILI) that disperse during the influenza season.

Influenza Virus Subtypes

The term 'flu' is used for almost any respiratory illness with systemic disorders, which might be caused by a plethora of viral or bacterial agents in addition to influenza viruses. But, true flu is a serious infectious disease brought on by a member of the orthomyxovirus family, including influenza viruses A, B, and C. Influenza outbreaks generally occur in winter in temperate climates. In the USA, the flu season starts in October or November and peaks between March and December. Important outbreaks of flu are connected with influenza virus type A or B. Influenza A infects birds, people, swine, horses, dogs, and seals. Influenza A is accountable for regular, generally annual outbreaks or epidemics of varying seriousness, and intermittent pandemics, whereas influenza B triggers outbreaks each two to four decades. Influenza B viruses create exactly the identical spectrum of disease as influenza A. However, influenza B viruses don't cause pandemics, maybe because they mostly infect people and rarely infect animals. Nearly all adults are infected with the influenza C virus, which induces respiratory tract disease that was moderate. Lower respiratory tract infections are infrequent.

Flu viruses are Classified with the following advice:

- Form A, B or C/place isolated/number of all

isolate/year isolated

• Influenza A is split into subtypes based on their hemagglutinin (H) and neuraminidase (N) proteins. There are 16 H and 9 N variations, but every virus has just 1 H and an N variation.

The influenza virus is an enveloped virus, meaning that the outer layer is a lipid membrane which the virus acquires from the host cell. Inserted into the lipid membrane will be the viral glycoprotein, hemagglutinin (H) and neuraminidase (N). Influenza A virions have three membrane proteins (H, N, and M2), whilst Influenza B virions have four (H, N, NB, and BM2). Under the lipid membrane is your M1 viral matrix protein that offers strength and rigidity into the viral envelope. The M2 protein is a proton station that's the goal of these antiviral drugs amantadine and rimantadine. Within influenza, B, or A virion are eight sections of viral RNA that take all of the genetic information required to synthesize new virus contamination. These RNA sections are tagged HA (hemagglutinin), NA (neuraminidase), PB1, PB2, PA, NP, M, and NS. Antigens on the inner proteins M1 and NP are type-specific and utilized to ascertain whether a specific flu virus is type A, B, or C. The two M1 and NP proteins of members of every kind display cross reactivity. Hemagglutinin is a surface glycoprotein that binds to sialic acid residues to epithelial cell surface glycoprotein. This interaction is essential for attachment and fusion of viral and cell membranes that are senile. Neuraminidase digests sialic acid (neuraminic acid) on the surface of cells, boosting entry of the virus to the cell. Neuraminidase facilitates penetration of the mucous coating in the lymph nodes. By late disease, virtually all sialic acid was taken away from infected cell surface, which makes it is simpler to get progeny virions to disseminate to other tissues. N is the goal of these anti-inflammatory drugs Relenza and Tamiflu.

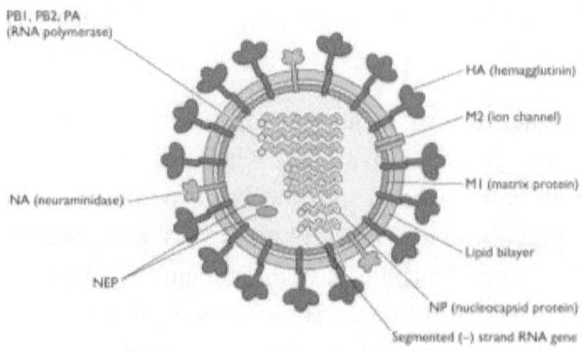

Influenza C viruses tend to be somewhat distinct. They contain 7 RNA segments rather than eight. The significant influenza C virus glycoprotein is known as HEF (hemagglutinin-esterase-fusion) since it has the functions of both the N and H. A small viral envelope protein is CM2, which acts as an ion channel. N and H display more antigenic variation compared to inner proteins and would be the significant determinants of both Influenza A subtype along with strain-specificity. Together with 16 H and 9 N, you will find 144 potential subtypes of influenza A. Minor changes in the envelope glycoprotein, hemagglutinin, and neuraminidase, are known as antigenic drift, and significant changes are known as antigenic shifts. Antigenic drifts are connected with localized outbreaks, while antigenic changes are correlated with epidemics and pandemics of Influenza A. Antigenic drift is because of a point mutation at HA or NA. Inefficient proofreading by Influenza viral RNA polymerase leads to a high prevalence of transcription mistakes and amino acid substitutions from hemagglutinin or neuraminidase, enabling new versions to prevent preexisting humoral resistance and lead to Influenza outbreaks. An individual resistant to the initial strain isn't resistant to the drifted one. The antigenic shift is because of HA or NA gene reassortment which ends in the synthesis of H or N protein variations. Wild birds are the natural hosts of influenza A virus, for many subtypes. Pigs also play an essential part in the growth of human pandemic strains since pig trachea comprises receptors for both avian and human influenza viruses, and reptiles encourage the development of both kinds of viruses. Genetic reassortment between avian and human virus might occur in cows, resulting in a novel strain. When a pig gets infected with both human and avian viruses, then the RNAs of both viruses have been duplicated in the nucleus. When new virus particles are constructed in the cell membrane, a number of these RNA segments can arise from both of the infecting viruses. New viruses that inherit RNA from the avian and human flu are known as reassortants. They may comprise creature and human proteins H or N. Whether this virus reassortant can infect people, they are going to have little resistance to it, raising the odds of an outbreak or pandemic. The H1N1 pandemic, which happened in 2009, was because of the reassortment of avian, human, and swine influenza viruses.

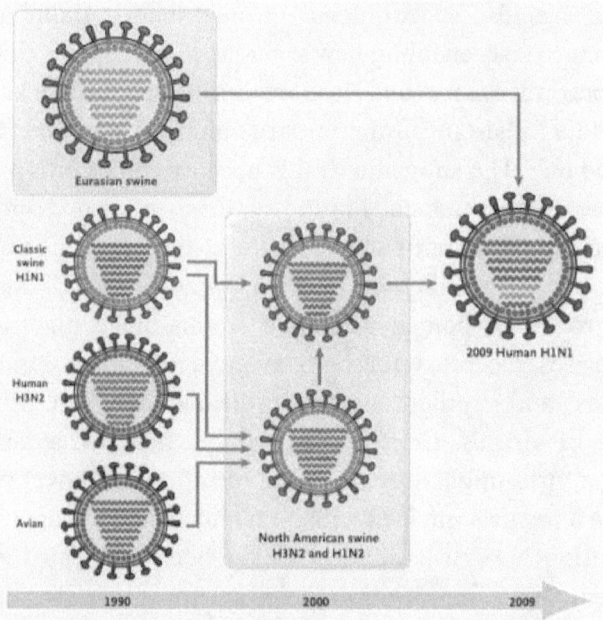

Reassortment can happen between influenza viruses of this same kind. Why influenza A viruses never swap RNA sections with influenza B or B 18 isn't known. Influenza B is not as prone to undergo antigenic change because there's not an animal reservoir for this virus.

Human Influenza

Even though nine N virus subtypes and 16 H happen in their Natural reservoir of aquatic creatures, just three hemagglutinin subtypes (H1, H2, and H3) and two neuraminidase subtypes (N1 and N2) have demonstrated stable lineages in people and generated widespread human respiratory disease. Today H3N2 and h1N1 cause epidemics. Changes have been responsible. The extremely severe outbreak of 1918 and 1919 (swine flu or Spanish flu) has been connected with the development of antigenic changes in both hemagglutinin (H1) and neuraminidase (N1) of influenza A. Between 50 and 100 million people were killed by this virus. The H1N1 virus responsible was derived from an avian strain that adapted to infect and efficiently transmit between humans. A lot of flu pandemics have occurred throughout the 20th century in people. In 1957, a change was made by a reassortant. This virus has been known as influenza since it originated in China and then spread worldwide. It caused between 4 and 1 million deaths and continued until 1958. Back in 1968, another human-avian reassortant generated an antigenic change from H2N2 into H3N2 (Hong Kong flu). Considering that the change involved hemagglutinin, this outbreak was less extensive, inducing 750,000 deaths. H3N2 influenza A reoccurred in 2006 and late 2003. It's now endemic in both pig and individual populations. The resistance to the virus has risen from 1 percent in 1994.

In 1977, an influenza A was generated by people who lacked preexisting resistance were influenced by that to H1N1. Since the late 1990s, reassortant swine influenza, A virus genes from swine, human, and avian strains of influenza, have been detected among swine herds in North America. Back in an epidemic of H1N1, March 2009 Influenza A virus has been discovered in Mexico that propagates States, Canada, and the world. The pandemic was announced to be over in August 2010. A reassortment of 2 caused this pandemic. Strains that are swine, one anxiety that is human, and yet another avian strain of influenza. The virus was known as Swine Flu since the proportion of genes originated from swine Influenza viruses. In reaction to this possibility of a pandemic, a vaccination campaign employing a monovalent vaccine has been undertaken. Even though The WHO announced that this pandemic over this H1N1 strain proceeds to circulate around the world together with influenza. H1N1 was comprised of the influenza vaccine that is 2011. Influenza A viruses, which people may be infected by circulating in creatures. These germs are known to as "version influenza viruses" and, as an abbreviation, will be designated using a "v." As of December 23, 2011, the Centers for Disease Control and Prevention (CDC) has received reports of 35 instances of human disease with esophageal origin variant flu viruses since 2005. The frequency with which these variant influenza viruses have been detected has increased since 2011. In the past 6 months of 2011, 12 US inhabitants in five distinct countries (Indiana, Iowa, Maine, Pennsylvania, and West Virginia) have been discovered to be infected with this specific influenza A version virus, which had genes in human flu, swine, and avian viruses. This virus differs from the other cases because it has acquired another genetic change, the matrix (M) gene from the 2009 H1N1 pandemic virus. Currently, nobody knows what the M gene's accession means in relation to disease severity or transmissibility in humans. So far, sickness associated with this particular virus has been self-limited and light. Restricted serologic studies conducted at CDC imply that adults might have some preexisting resistance to H3N2v kids don't. The next diagram demonstrates how the virus generated from the reassortment of this matrix. (M) Gene segments in the 2009 H1N1 virus that is pandemic using the HA and NA gene Segments in the Swine H3N2 reassortment virus in 1998 -- 2011.

Construction And Genetics

Influenza type A viruses are extremely similar in construction to Influenza viruses forms B, C, and D. The virus particle (also referred to as the virion) is 80-120 nanometers in diameter like the tiniest virions embrace an elliptical form. Every particle's duration may be in excess of thousands of micrometers, making virions, and fluctuates because of the fact that flu is Pleomorphic. Confusion regarding the nature of the Influenza virus pleomorphic originates from the observation that laboratory-adapted strains normally decrease the ability to make filaments and these laboratory-adapted strains were the first to be visualized by electron microscopy. Despite these shapes, viruses are similar in makeup. They're all composed of an envelope comprising two kinds of proteins. Both big proteins found in the exterior of viral contaminants are hemagglutinin (HA) and neuraminidase (NA). HA is a protein that mediates the binding of the virion to the target entrance and cells of the viral genome. NA is included in discharge in the abundant attachment websites within mucus in addition to the release of virions from cells that were infected. These proteins are the targets for drugs. Furthermore, they are also the antigen proteins to which a host's antibodies can bind and trigger an immune response. Influenza type A viruses have been categorized into subtypes based on the face of the envelope. You will find 9 subtypes of NA understood and 16 subtypes of HA, but H 1, 3, and 2, and N 2 and 1 are found in people. The core of a virion includes other proteins that protect and pack the material and the genome. Unlike the genomes of most organisms (such as humans, plants, animals, and bacteria) that are composed of double-stranded DNA, several viral genomes comprise another, single-stranded nucleic acid known as RNA. Unusually for a virus the influenza type A virus genome isn't a single bit of RNA, but rather, it is composed of segmented parts of negative-sense RNA: every piece comprising either a couple of genes that code for a gene product (protein). The expression negative-sense RNA just suggests the RNA genome cannot be translated into protein straight; it should first be transcribed to positive-sense RNA before it can be translated into protein solutions. The nature of the genome allows for the exchange of genes between different strains.

The entire Influenza A virus genome is 13,588 bases long and is contained on eight RNA segments that code for at least 10 but up to 14 proteins, depending on the strain. The significance of the existence of alternative gene products may differ:

•   Segment 1 encodes RNA polymerase subunit (PB2).

•   Segment 2 Fragrant RNA polymerase subunit (PB1) and also the PB1-F2 protein, which induces cell death, using different reading frames from precisely the exact same RNA segment.

•   Segment 3 encodes RNA polymerase subunit (PA) and the PA-X protein, which has a role in host transcription shutoff.

•   Segment 4 encodes for HA (hemagglutinin). Approximately 500 molecules of hemagglutinin are essential to creating 1 virion. HA determines the seriousness and the scope of a viral disease in a host organism.

•   Segment 5 encodes NP, which is a nucleoprotein.

- Segment 6 encodes NA (neuraminidase). Approximately 100 molecules of neuraminidase are essential to creating 1 virion.

- Segment 7 encodes two matrix proteins (M1 and M2) using different reading frames from precisely the exact same RNA segment. About 3,000 matrix protein molecules are essential to creating 1 virion.

- Segment 8 encodes two different non-structural proteins (NS1 and NEP) using different reading frames from precisely the exact same RNA segment.

The RNA segments of the genome have foundation sequences in the terminal endings, letting them bond. Transcription of the viral (-) sense genome (v RNA) can only move following the PB2 protein binds to host restricted RNAs, allowing for the PA subunit to cleave several nucleotides following the cap. This cap and nucleotides that are accompanied function as the primer for transcription initiation. Transcription proceeds across the vRNA before a stretch of many Uralic bases is attained, initiating a 'stuttering' where the viral mRNA is poly-adenylated, making a mature transcript for nuclear export and translation by sponsor machines. While the synthesis of proteins occurs in the cytoplasm, the RNA synthesis occurs from the cell nucleus. When the viral proteins have been built into virions, the constructed virions leave the nucleus and migrate to the cell membrane. [32] The host cell membrane contains stains of viral transmembrane proteins (HA, NA, and M2) and an underlying layer of the M1 protein that helps the constructed virions to bud throughout the membrane, releasing completed enveloped viruses to the extracellular fluid.

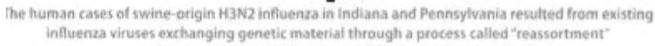

The human cases of swine-origin H3N2 influenza in Indiana and Pennsylvania resulted from existing influenza viruses exchanging genetic material through a process called "reassortment"

(Influenza A viruses have 8 RNA segments: HA, NA, PB1, PB2, PA, NP, M, NS)

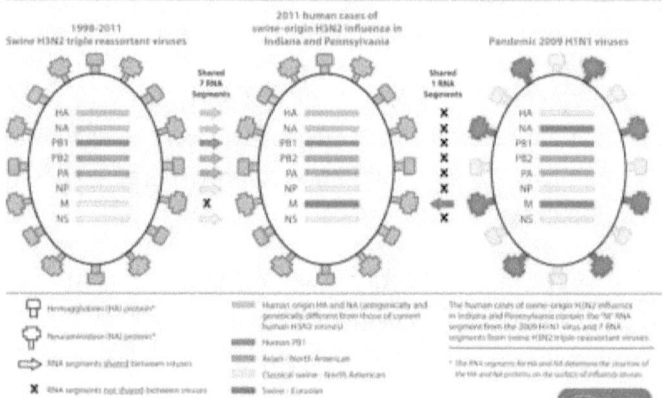

Influenza A (H3N2) v viruses discovered thus far are vulnerable Into oseltamivir (Tamiflu®) or zanamivir (Relenza®). As these viruses possess the gene in the influenza A (H1N1) pdm09 virus, they are resistant to amantadine and rimantadine.

Avian Influenza

Viruses that infect domestic or wild birds Cause limited illness. But, properties that have made them more virulent have been obtained by viruses inside the H5 and H7 subtypes. Avian H5N1 influenza A viruses have been endemic among poultry and bird populations, and therefore are regarded as the world's leading flu pandemic threat. The primary institution of avian influenza H5N1 with clinical respiratory disease happened in Hong Kong in 1997 through a poultry epidemic of highly pathogenic H5N1 flu in live-bird markets. This epidemic was associated with a mortality rate and a high prevalence of pneumonia. All virus genes were indicating that the species barrier had jumped. Surveillance showed evidence of transmission, and no cases were reported after the culling of poultry. Since its development in humans in 1997, influenza H5N1 has experienced antigenic drift. H5N1 virus seems to have expanded its host array besides infecting humans and poultry. Fatal disease in cats was reported. There are no reports of cats distributing the virus. All human H5 infections have caused viruses to own the subtype. Concern remains that this strain may mutate, or experience reassortment and get the ability to spread from human to human. Avian influenza H7 viruses also have been associated with the disorder that was occasional. Subtype H7 viruses with numerous N subtypes (N2, N3, and N7) have transmitted from birds to people. Outbreaks of H7N7 occurred among poultry in the Netherlands. Employees had grown influenza-like disease and conjunctivitis. Infections are reported among poultry workers in Italy, the USA, Canada, and the United Kingdom. Much like H5N1, all genes in the viruses have been avian in origin. Avian H9N2 viruses are endemic in poultry in Asia and are isolated from cows. By kids with moderate respiratory disease, influenza H9N2 viruses have been isolated back in Hong Kong in 1999, 2003, 2007, and 2009. The viruses are responsible for the 1999 ailments comprised enzymes homologous, implying that these strains roseby reassortment.

Kinds Of Flu

Not all influenza areequal. Some forms can make you quite sick, though milder symptoms are caused by other kinds of influenza. Keep reading to learn about different kinds of flu.

How Can A Flu Virus Make Me Sick?

Flu viruses enter the body through your nose, mouth, or eyes. Every time you touch your hands you're possibly infecting yourself. This makes it important to keep your palms virus-free with thorough and regular hand washing. Advise relatives to do the exact same to protect against the flu.

What Are The Different Types Of Flu?

There are 3 Kinds of influenza viruses: A, B, and C. Type A And B trigger the yearly flu epidemics, which have around 20 percent of the populace sniffling, coughing, and conducting high fevers. Form C also causes influenza. Type C influenza symptoms are not as severe. The flu is related to 49,000 deaths and between 3,000 and 200,000 hospitalizations every year. The influenza vaccine was produced to attempt and prevent these epidemics.

What's Type A Flu?

Type influenza or flu Animals, even though it is common for individuals to endure the ailments related to this kind of flu. Wild birds act as hosts because of this particular flu virus. Type A influenza virus is continually changing and is normally responsible for the huge flu epidemics. The influenza A2 virus (along with other forms of flu) is spread by those that are infected. The most common flu hot spots are those surfaces that an infected person has touched and rooms where he or she has been recently, especially areas where he or she has been sneezing.

What's Type B Flu? Type B influenza is located in

humans. Type B influenza might cause a less intense response than type A influenza virus, but sometimes type B influenza may still be extremely dangerous. Influenza type B viruses aren't categorized by subtype and don't cause pandemics.

How Is Type C Flu Virus Different From Others?

Influenza C viruses are found in humans. They're milder than type A or B. People do not become very ill in the flu type C viruses. Type C influenza viruses cause epidemics that do not cause epidemics.

Do Different Kinds Of Flu Viruses Reach The Population Every Year?

Various strains of influenza replace the strains of this virus. That is the reason it's important to have a flu shot every year to make sure your entire body develops resistance to the latest strains of this virus. According to the CDC, the viruses at a flu shot and Flu Mist vaccine may change annually based on international surveillance and scientists' estimations about which types and strains of influenza will probably be potent annually. Formerly, all influenza vaccines protected against three flu viruses: 1 Influenza A (H3N2) virus, 1 Influenza A (H1N1) virus, and one Influenza B virus. Now, Flu Mist, plus a few conventional flu shots, normally cover around four strains: 2 Influenza A viruses along with 2 Influenza B viruses. Approximately two weeks after having a flu shot or Flu Mist, antibodies that provide protection from the influenza viruses grow inside the human body. Nevertheless, Flu Mist is also not suggested for use throughout the 2017-2018 season since it may not be powerful.

What's The Bird Flu?

Bird flu is caused by the influenza virus. Birds can be infected by all its subtypes and influenza A viruses. Birds aren't capable of carrying type C or B flu viruses. There are three subtypes of avian influenza. Even the subtypes H5 and H7 are the most deadly, although the H9 subtype is not as dangerous.

Which Kind Of Bird Flu Is In The News?

Health care professionals were quite vocal regarding the strain of avian influenza called H5N1. The main reason H5N1 has caused so much alarm is the way it can maneuver from wild birds to poultry, then on to individuals. While wild birds are generally resistant to the catastrophic and potentially deadly consequences of H5N1, the virus has killed over half of those people infected with it. The possibility of avian flu is usually low in the majority of people since the virus doesn't normally infect humans. Infections have occurred as the result of contact with infected birds. The spread of the disease from humans to humans has been reported to be quite rare.

Should I Understand Catching Bird Flu?

Individuals in the USA have less to fear than individuals who live overseas. The majority of the illnesses have been reported among those who've had contact with farm animals in nations. Additionally, individuals aren't able to capture the bird influenza virus from eating cooked chicken, turkey, or duck. The virus is killed by high temperatures.

Is There A Vaccine For Bird Flu?

No. It's crucial that you know the influenza vaccine doesn't offer protection against bird flu or avian flu.

Influenza Type A Viruses

There are four kinds of influenza viruses: A, B, C, and D. Wild aquatic birds -- especially specific wild ducks, geese, swans, gulls, shorebirds and terns -- would be the natural hosts for many flu types A viruses.

Subtypes Of Influenza A Infection

Influenza A viruses are divided into subtypes on the basis of two proteins on the surface of the virus: hemagglutinin (HA) and neuraminidase (NA). There are 11 NA subtypes and 18 known HA subtypes. Many distinct combinations of HA and NA proteins are possible. For example, an "H7N2 virus" designates the influenza A virus subtype that has an HA 7 protein and an NA two protein. In the same way, an "H5N1" virus has an HA 5 protein and an NA 1 protein. All known subtypes of influenza A viruses can infect birds, except subtypes H17N10 and H18N11; that has just been discovered in rodents. Just two influenza A virus subtypes (i.e., H1N1, and H3N2) are now in general circulation among individuals. Some subtypes are located in animal species that were contaminated. Some subtypes are found in other infected animal species. For example, H7N7 and H3N8 virus infections can cause illness in horses, and H3N8 virus infection causes illness in horses and dogs.

Lineages Of Influenza A Infection

Avian influenza (AI) viruses – influenza viruses that infect birds – have evolved into distinct genetic lineages in different geographic locations. These various lineages may be distinguished by analyzing the hereditary make-up of those viruses. By way of instance, AI viruses circulating in birds from Asia, known as Oriental lineage AI viruses, could be considered genetically distinct from AI viruses that circulate among birds in North America (known as North American lineage AI viruses). These wide lineage classifications could be further narrowed by genetic comparisons that enable researchers to set the many closely-related viruses collectively. Therefore, the North American lineage of all H7N9 viruses might be further broken down to the North American 'wild bird' lineage versus the North American 'poultry' lineage. The hosts, time period, and geographic location are frequently utilized in the lineage title to assist further delineate 1 lineage from the other.

Highly Pathogenic And Low Pathogenic Avian Influenza A Viruses

Avian flu A viruses have been designated as highly pathogenic avian influenza (HPAI) or very low pathogenicity avian influenza (LPAI) based on molecular features of the virus and the capability of the virus to cause illness and mortality in cows at a lab setting. HPAI and LPAI designations don't refer to the seriousness of the disease in cases of human infection with these viruses; both LPAI and HPAI viruses have caused acute illness in humans. Poultry infected with LPAI viruses might show no symptoms of a disorder or just exhibit mild illness (such as ruffled feathers and a drop in egg production) that might not be discovered. The infection of poultry together with HPAI viruses can result in severe illness. The two LPAI and HPAI viruses could propagate quickly through poultry flocks. HPAI virus disease can lead to disease that affects multiple internal organs together with mortality around 90% to 100% in cows, often within two days. Ducks may be infected with no symptoms of illness. There are genetic and antigenic differences between the flu A virus subtypes that normally infect creatures and the ones that could infect birds and humans. Avian flu viruses infect individuals. The most often identified subtypes of avian flu that have caused human infections are H5, H7, and H9 viruses. Other viruses, such as H10N8, H10N7, and H6N8, are discovered in humans but to a lesser degree.

Influenza A H5

There are known subtypes of H5 (H5N1, H5N2, H5N3, H5N4, H5N5, H5N6, H5N7, H5N8, and H5N9). Many H5 viruses found globally in wild fish and birds are LPAI, but sometimes HPAI viruses are detected. A sporadic H5 virus disease of people has happened, for example, with Asian lineage because HPAI H5N1 viruses are now circulating among poultry in Asia and the Middle East. Human infection of H5N1 virus infections is reported in 16 states, often leading to acute pneumonia and higher than 50% mortality.

Influenza A H7

There are known subtypes of (H7N1, H7N2, H7N3, H7N4, H7N5, H7N6, H7N7, H7N8, and H7N9). H7 viruses found in wild fish and birds are LPAI viruses. Virus disease in humans is rare. The most often identified H7 viruses associated with human disease are lineage avian influenza A (H7N9) viruses, which have been detected in China in 2013. While human infections are infrequent, these have resulted in acute respiratory illness and passing. Along with Asian H7N9 viruses, H7N7 virus diseases are reported. These viruses have mostly induced mild to moderate illness in humans, with symptoms that have conjunctivitis or upper respiratory tract ailments.

Influenza A H9

There are known subtypes of H9 (H9N1, H9N2, H9N3, H9N4, H9N5, H9N6, H9N7, H9N8, and H9N9); all of the H9 viruses identified globally in wild fish and birds are LPAI viruses. The virus has been found in bird populations in Africa, Europe, the Middle East, and Asia. Unusual, intermittent H9N2 virus infections in people are reported to normally cause mild upper respiratory tract disease; one disease has led to death.

Chapter - 6 The Flu Season

While seasonal influenza (flu) viruses have been detected year-round in the USA, influenza viruses are most frequent during winter and the autumn. Flu activity starts to rise in October, although the time and duration of influenza seasons may vary. Most of the time flu activity peaks between December and February, although activity can last as late as May. The figure below reveals flu action in the United States. The "peak month of flu activity" is the month with the highest percentage of respiratory specimens testing positive for influenza virus infection during that influenza season. During this 36-year period, flu activity most often peaked in February (15 seasons), followed by December (7 seasons), January (6 seasons), and March (6 seasons).

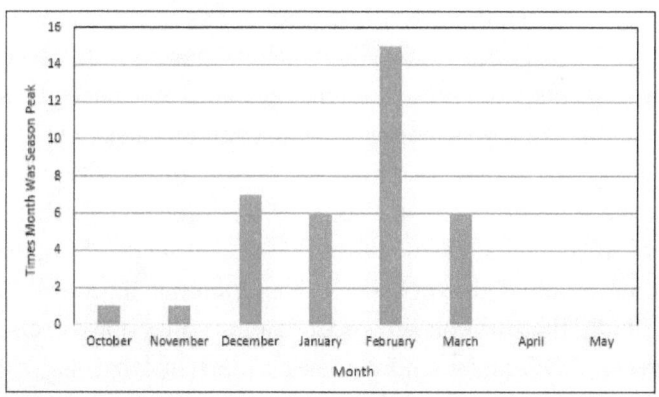

When Is The Flu Season In The USA?

In the USA, flu season happens in the autumn and winter. While flu viruses circulate year-round, the majority of the time influenza action peaks between February and December, however, action can last as late as May. The general health impact (e.g., infections, hospitalizations, and deaths) of a flu season fluctuates from season to season. CDC collects, compiles, and analyzes information on flu action year-long in the USA and generates Flu View, a weekly surveillance report, and Flu View Interactive, allowing for much more in-depth exploration of flu surveillance information. The Weekly U.S. Influenza Summary Update is updated each week from October through May.

How Can CDC Track The Development Of The Influenza Season?

The general health impact (e.g., infections, hospitalizations, and deaths) of a flu season fluctuates from season to season. CDC collects, compiles, and analyzes data on a surveillance report flu action yearlong in the USA and produces FluView, a weekly surveillance report, and FluView Interactive, which allows for a more in-depth exploration of influenza surveillance data. The Weekly U.S. Influenza Summary Update is updated every week from October through May. The U.S. flu surveillance process is a collaborative effort between CDC and its numerous partners in local and state health departments, public health and medical labs, vital statistics offices, healthcare providers, and practices and emergency departments. Info in five classes is gathered from eight Distinct data sources which enable CDC to:

- Learn where and when influenza activity is happening

- Track influenza-related disease

- Determine what flu viruses have been circulating

- Detect changes in flu viruses

- Assess the impact the flu is having to hospitalizations and deaths from the USA

These surveillance elements allow CDC to determine if and where influenza activity is currently happening, determine what kinds of flu viruses are currently circulating, detect changes in the flu viruses examined and collected, assess the effect of flu, and monitor patterns of disease. All influenza activity reporting by states, laboratories, and health care providers is voluntary. For more information about CDC's influenza surveillance activities, see the Overview of Influenza Surveillance in the United States.

Why Can There Be A Week-Long Lag Between The Information And As Soon As It's Documented?

Influenza surveillance information collection relies on a reporting. It starts on Sunday and ends on the Saturday of every week. Each surveillance player is asked to outline the information that was weekly and submit an application to the CDC. The data is downloaded, compiled, and analyzed in the CDC. The data is utilized to upgrade Flu View Interactive and FluView.

Do Other Respiratory Viruses Circulate Throughout The Influenza Season?

In addition to flu viruses, several other respiratory viruses also circulate during the flu season and can cause symptoms and illnesses similar to those seen with flu infection. These respiratory viruses comprise rhinovirus (one reason for this "common cold") and respiratory syncytial virus (RSV), that's the usual cause of acute respiratory disease in young children, in addition to a chief cause of death from respiratory disease in people aged 65 years and older.

When Exactly Is Flu Season?

Although flu season is usually thought of as occurring in the winter, the severity and timing vary from year to year. To best protect you no matter the particular interval, the Centers for Disease Control and Prevention (CDC) recommends getting vaccinated at the end of October.

In general, flu season in the United States can start anytime in late fall, peak in mid-to-late winter (between December and February), and continue through early spring. Flu season lasts about 13 weeks. In a few years it could linger into May, although it is going to finish by April. It's a great idea you receivev the flu shot, but a late influenza shot offers protection when flu season descends into April or even May.

Check Out Past Flu Seasons

The strain of flu that circulates can change from year to year, and the vaccine is adjusted in an attempt to predict which will predominate. Here's a look at the flu within the last 10 years:

2018-2019 Flu Seasons:

- Peak: Mid-February

- Most Frequent strain: Influenza A--both H3N2 and H1N1

2017-2018 Flu Seasons:

- Peak: January and February

- Most Frequent strain: Influenza A (H3N2)

2016-2017 Flu Seasons:

- Peak: Mid-March

- Most Frequent strain: Influenza A (H3N2)

2015-2016 Flu Seasons:

- Peak: Mid-March

- Most Frequent strain: 2009 H1N1 Influenza A

2014-2015 Flu Seasons:

- Peak: overdue December

- Most Frequent strain: Influenza A (H3N2)

2013-2014 Flu Seasons:

- Peak: overdue December

- Most Frequent strain: 2009 H1N1 Influenza A

2012-2013 Flu Seasons:

- Peak: overdue December

- Most Frequent strain: Influenza A (H3N2)

2011-2012 Flu Seasons:

- Peak: Mid-March

- Most Frequent strain: Influenza A (H3N2)

2010-2011 Flu Seasons:

- Peak: Historical February

- Most Frequent strain: Influenza A (H3N2)

Cause

Three virus families, Influenza virus A, B, and C, are the main infective agents that cause influenza. During periods of temperatures, flu cases grow. Despite the higher incidence of manifestations of the flu during the season, the viruses are actually transmitted throughout populations all year round. Every yearly flu season is generally connected with a significant influenza virus subtype. The related subtype affects every year because of the growth of immunological resistance to some preceding year's strain (through vaccinations and vulnerability), and mutational changes in formerly dormant viruses strains.

The Precise mechanism Supporting the character of flu outbreaks is unknown. Some suggested explanations are:

- Individuals are indoors more often during the winter, they are in close contact more often, and this promotes transmission from person to person.

• A seasonal decrease in the quantity of ultraviolet radiation can lessen the probability of the virus being ruined or damaged by direct radiation harm or indirect consequences (i.e. ozone concentration), increasing the probability of infection.

• Cold temperatures contribute to the drier atmosphere, which may dehydrate mucous membranes, preventing the body from effectively defending against respiratory virus infections.

• Viruses are maintained in colder temperatures because of slower decomposition, allowing them to linger longer on exposed surfaces (doorknobs, countertops, etc.).

• In countries where children do not go to school in the summer, there is a more pronounced beginning to flu season, coinciding with the start of public school. [citation needed] It is thought that the daycare environment is perfect for the spread of illness.

• Vitamin D production by Ultraviolet-B from skin impacts the immune system also varies with the seasons.

Research in guinea pigs has shown that the aerosol transmission of the virus is enhanced when the air is cold and dry. The dependence on aridity seems to be a result of degradation of the virus contamination in the atmosphere, while the dependence on chilly appears to be attributed to hosts losing the virus. The investigators didn't find the chilly impaired the guinea pigs' reaction. Research performed by the National Institute of Child Health and Human

Development (NICHD) in 2008 discovered that the flu virus has a "butter-like Coating." As it passes the lymph nodes, the coat melts. From the coat becomes a shell. In winter, it can survive in the cold weather very similar to a spore. In the summer, the coating melts before the virus reaches the respiratory tract.

Flu Vaccinations

Flu vaccinations have been used to reduce the effects of the influenza season. Pneumonia vaccinations diminish complications and the ramifications of the influenza season. Since the Northern and Southern Hemisphere has wintered at different times of the year, there are actually two flu seasons each year. Hence, the World Health Organization (aided by the National Influenza Centers) makes two vaccine formulations every year; just one to the Northern, and one to the Southern Hemisphere.

According to the U.S. Department of Health, a growing amount of large businesses provide their workers with seasonal influenza shots, either with a little cost to the worker or as a totally free service. The yearly updated trivalent flu vaccine includes hemagglutinin (HA) surface glycoprotein elements from influenza H3N2, H1N1, and B flu viruses. The strain in January 2006 has been H3N2. Measured resistance to the standard antiviral drugs amantadine and rimantadine in H3N2 has increased from 1% in 1994 to 12% in 2003 to 91% in 2005.

Associated Health Issues

Medical conditions that compromise the immune system

increase the risks of flu.

Diabetes

Huge numbers of individuals have diabetes. When blood sugars aren't controlled, diabetics may create a broad variety of complications. Diabetes contributes to elevated blood sugars within the human body, and also this environment permits bacteria and viruses to flourish. If blood sugars have been poorly controlled, moderate flu can easily turn acute, resulting in illness and even death. Uncontrolled blood sugars suppress the immune systems and generally lead to more severe cases of the common cold or influenza. It has been advocated that diabetics have been vaccinated against influenza before the start of the flu season.

Asthma/COPD

It's suggested that asthmatics and COPD patients be vaccinated before the influenza season against influenza. People with asthma may create complications from common cold viruses and flu. Some of the complications include acute respiratory distress syndrome, severe bronchitis, and pneumonia. Every year influenza-related complications in the United States and countless more are observed in the emergency room because of shortness of breath. It's encouraged that asthmatics be vaccinated before the summit of the influenza season, between October and November. Flu vaccine requires about two weeks; it works by boosting the body's immune system.

Cancer

Individuals with cancer have a suppressed immune system.

Additionally, many cancer patients undergo radiation treatment and powerful immunosuppressive drugs, which additionally inhibits the body's ability to fight infections. Everybody with cancer can be at risk for complications from influenza and is vulnerable. People with cancer or a history of cancer should receive the seasonal flu shot. As cancer results in complications of hepatitis and pneumonia, the flu vaccination is rigorous for lung cancer sufferers. People with cancer shouldn't get the nasal spray medication. The flu shot is made up of inactivated (killed) viruses, and the nasal spray vaccines are made up of live viruses. The flu shot is much more powerful for people who have a diminished immune system. People who have received cancer treatment, like radiation or chemotherapy treatment over the previous month, or have a blood or lymphatic kind of cancer, must call their physician immediately if they suspect they might have flu.

Hiv/Aids

(HIV) are extremely prone to many different infections. HIV has a huge capability to destroy the human body's immune system and this makes one more prone to not only viral diseases but also fungal, bacterial, and protozoa ailments. People with HIV are at a heightened risk of severe complications. Reports have shown that people with HIV can create cases of pneumonia that require antibiotic treatment and hospitalization. People are at a higher risk of passing and with HIV have an influenza season that is lengthier. Vaccination using the flu shot was proven to increase the immune system and guard against seasonal influenza in certain patients with HIV; people who have HIV should just get vaccinated with the inactivated flu vaccine. Any HIV patient who has been exposed to other people with influenza should see a physician to determine if there is a need for anti-viral medications.

Price

The expense of a flu season in lives lost, medical expenses, and economic impact can be severe.

• "In the USA of America, for instance, recent estimates place the price of flu epidemics into the market at $71-167 billion US dollars annually."

A study estimated that in the United States, annual influenza epidemics result in approximately 600,000 life-years lost, 3 million hospitalized days, and 30 million outpatient visits, resulting in medical costs of $10 billion annually. According to the research, lost earnings due to sickness and loss of life amounted to over $15 billion annually and the overall financial burden of annual flu epidemics figures to over $80 billion. In addition, in the US, the influenza season generally accounts for 200,000 hospitalizations and 41,000 deaths. Since the mortality rate of this H1N1 "swine flu" is significantly lower compared to influenza strains, this amount was reduced in 2009. Based on an article in Clinical Infectious Diseases, printed in 2011, the estimated health burden of 2009 Pandemic Influenza A (H1N1), between April 2009 to April 2010, has been "roughly 60.8 million cases (array: 43.3--89.3 million), 274,304 hospitalizations (195,086--402,719), along with 12,469 deaths (8,868--18,306)" at the USA because of pH1N1."

How Flu Spreads

Person To Person

It can be spread by Individuals with influenza to other people around approximately 6 ft away. Experts believe influenza viruses spread by droplets created when individuals speak, cough, or sneeze. These droplets can land in the mouths or noses of people who are nearby or possibly be inhaled into the lungs. Less often, a person might get the flu by touching a surface or object that has the flu virus on it and then touching their own mouth, nose, or possibly their eyes.

When Flu Spread

Individuals with influenza are contagious in the first three to four days after their illness starts. Most healthy adults may have the ability to infect others beginning 1 day before symptoms develop and up to 5 to 7 days after getting ill. A few individuals with weakened immune systems and kids can pass the virus. Symptoms may start about two times (but may vary from 1 to 4 times) after the virus enters your system. That usually means you might have the ability to pass on the flu to someone else before you know you're sick or while sick. Some people can be infected with the flu virus but have no signs. Those individuals may spread the virus.

Stage Of Contagiousness

You may have the ability to pass the flu to someone else before you understand you're sick.

•   Individuals with influenza are contagious in the first 3-4 days after their illness starts

•   Some otherwise healthy adults may have the ability

to infect others beginning 1 day before symptoms develop and up to 5 to 7 days after getting ill

•   Some individuals, particularly young children and individuals with weakened immune systems, may have the ability to infect other people with influenza viruses for an even longer time

Chapter - 7 Spanish Influenza (1918-20): The International Effect Of The Most Significant Flu Pandemic In History

In the past 150 years, the entire world has witnessed unprecedented improvement in wellbeing. The research indicates that in most countries life expectancy, which affects the average age of death, doubled from approximately 40 decades or less to over 80 decades. This wasn't only an accomplishment across these states. Life expectancy has doubled in most areas of the planet. What also stands out is how abrupt and damning negative health events can be. Most striking is that the large, sudden decrease of life expectancy in 1918 brought on by a remarkably deadly flu pandemic known as the famous 'Spanish flu.' To make sense of the fact that life expectancy declined so abruptly, one has to understand what it measures. Term life expectancy, that is the exact title for this step, just examines the mortality pattern in one specific year then catches this picture of public wellbeing as the average age of death using a hypothetical cohort of individuals so that year's mortality routine could stay constant throughout their whole lifetimes. Period life expectancy is a measure of their people's health in 1 year. This flu outbreak was not limited to Spain and it did not even arise there (a recent study from Olson et al. (2005) indicates that the outbreak originated from New York because of signs of a pre-pandemic tide of this virus in that town).

Nevertheless, it was called such because Spain was neutral in the First World War (1914-18), which meant it had been free to report the intensity of the outbreak, while nations which were fighting strove to curb reports how the flu affected their inhabitants to keep morale, not seem diminished in the opinion of the enemies. The flu outbreak began in the spring of 1918 from the Northern Hemisphere. The virus spread rapidly and eventually reached all parts of the world: the epidemic became a pandemic. In a much less-connected universe the virus finally reached extremely distant places like the Alaskan wilderness and Samoa at the center of the Pacific islands. While peak mortality was reached in 1918 the pandemic did not end until two years later in late 1920.

The International Death Count Of This Influenza Now

To have a circumstance for the severity of flu pandemics, it might be very helpful to be aware of the departure count of a normal flu season. Estimates for the number of deaths from the flu are approximately 400,000 deaths each year. Paget et al (2019) indicate a mean of 389,000 and having an uncertainty range 294,000 from 518,000.4 This implies that in the past few years, the flu has been responsible for the passing of 0.0052 percent of the world population -- just one individual for every 18,750.5 Even compared with the minimal quote because of the death count of Spanish influenza (17.4 million) this outbreak, over a century past, led to a death rate which has been 182 times greater than the current baseline. Further below I will briefly discuss similarities and differences with the Coronavirus (COVID-19) in 2019/20.

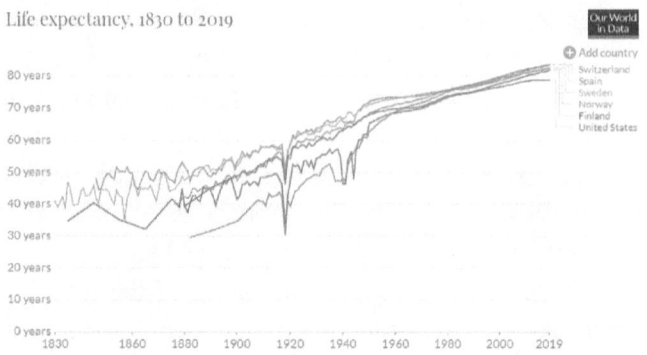

Life expectancy, 1830 to 2019

How Many People Died In The Spanish Flu And Other Influenza Pandemics?

Global Deaths Of The Spanish Influenza

Several research groups have worked on the issue that was challenging: reconstructing the health impact of this outbreak. There is now a lot of variability in these estimates and while the academic discussions continue, the range of estimates gives us an understanding of the severity of the event. The visualization here reveals the quotes that are available from the research book. Patterson and Pyle (1991) estimated that between 24.7 and 39.3 million died from the pandemic. The widely cited research by Johnson and Mueller (2002) arrives in a greater estimate of 50 million worldwide deaths. However, the authors suggest that this might be an underestimation and the real death toll was as large as 100 million. The recent analysis by Spreeuwenberg et al. (2018) reasoned that earlier estimates are too large. Their very own quote is 17.4 million deaths.

Global Death Rate

How do these estimates compare with the world's dimensions Population at the moment? How large was the share who died in the pandemic? Estimates imply that the world population in 1918 was 1.8 billion. According to this, the minimal estimate of 17.4 million deaths by Spreeuwenberg et al. (2018) suggests that Spanish influenza killed almost 1 percent (0.95percent) of the world population. If we rely upon the estimate of 50 million deaths released by Johnson and Mueller, it suggests that Spanish influenza killed 2.7 percent of the world population. And when it was actually high -- 100 million since those writers indicate -- then the worldwide death rate could have been 5.4percent. The entire population was rising by approximately 13 million annually in this interval, which suggests the length of the Spanish influenza was probably the last time ever once the world population was declining.

Other Big Flu Pandemics

The Spanish flu pandemic was the largest, but not the only large recent influenza pandemic. Two years before Spanish influenza the Russian influenza pandemic (1889-1894) is thought to have killed 1 million people. Estimates for its death toll of this "Asian Flu" (1957-1958) fluctuated between 1.5 and 4 million. Gatherer (2009) 13 published an estimate of 1.5 million, while Michaelis et al. (2009) published an estimate of two-4 million. Based on a WHO publication, the "Hong Kong Flu" (1968-1969) killed between 1 and 4 million individuals. Michaelis et al. (2009) released a lower estimate of 1-two million. The Russian Flu outbreak of 1977-78 was brought on by precisely the exact same H1N1 virus that caused the Spanish flu. In accordance with Michaelis et al. (2009), around 700,000 died worldwide. What becomes clear from this overview are two things: influenza pandemics are not rare, and the Spanish flu of 1918 was by far the most devastating influenza pandemic in recorded history.

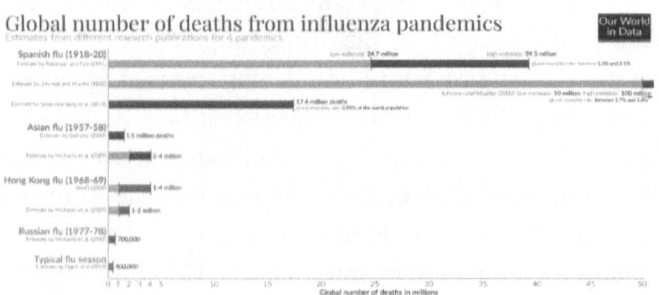

Global number of deaths from influenza pandemics

The Effect Of The Spanish Influenza Pandemic On Different Age Groups

This visualization shows the life expectancy in England and Wales by age. The red line indicates the life expectancy for a toddler, together with the lines for revealing how long a person could expect to live once they had reached that given, older, age. The green line, as an instance, signifies the life expectancy. It indicates that life expectancy improved at all ages, meaning the assertion that life expectancy 'just' improved because child mortality diminished isn't correct. This long-term rise of life expectancy at all ages is the focus of this accompanying text here. Related to the flu's effect, it's striking that the research demonstrates that the outbreak had little effect. Even though the life expectancy at ages and at birth dropped by over ten decades, the life expectancy of 60-70-year olds saw no modification. That is at odds with what we'd expect: people that are elderly are most vulnerable to ailments and flu outbreaks. If we take a look at mortality for lower respiratory infections (pneumonia) and upper respiratory ailments now, passing rates are greatest for people who are 70 decades and older. One reason why this pandemic was so devastating was that people accounted for a sizable share of the populace. Were individuals that are elderly resilient to the 1918 pandemic? The research literature indicates that this was true because elderly individuals had lived through a previous flu outbreak -- that the previously discussed 'Russian influenza pandemic' of 1889-90 -- which gave those who lived through it some immunity for the later outbreak of the Spanish flu. The earlier 1889-90 pandemic might have given the older population some immunity, but was a destructive event in itself. According to Smith, 132,000 people died in England, Wales, and Ireland alone.

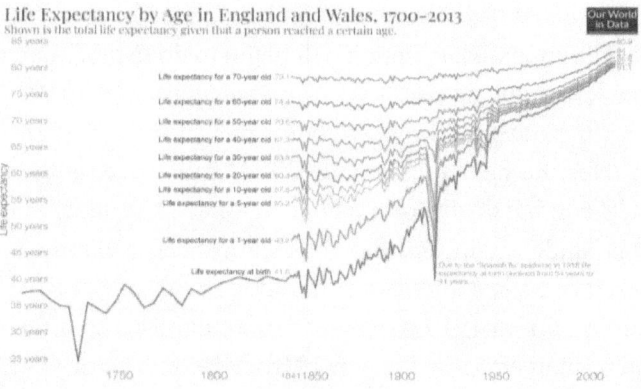

The Lasting Effects Of The 1918 Influenza Pandemic

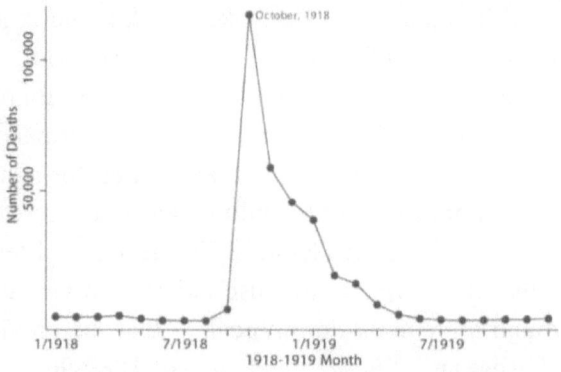

FIG. 1.—U.S. influenza deaths: *a*, by year; *b*, by month

I've never put a trigger warning on a post before, but given the current situation, the information here is potentially upsetting to anyone expecting a kid. I don't really feel the present pandemic will probably be as bad as 1918. I am optimistic that the weather will probably operate in our favor, as Tyler contended, America will begin to do the job. Do read my article, What amuses to get a message in 1918-1919? The 1918 flu pandemic struck ferocity in October of 1918 and then over the next four months killed more people than all the US combat deaths of the 20th century. The sudden nature of the pandemic meant that children born just months apart experienced very different conditions in utero. Specifically, children born in 1919 were much more exposed to influenza in utero than children born in 1918 or 1920. The differential to the 1918 flu allows in Is the 1918 Influenza Pandemic Over Douglas Almond test for consequences that are long-term.

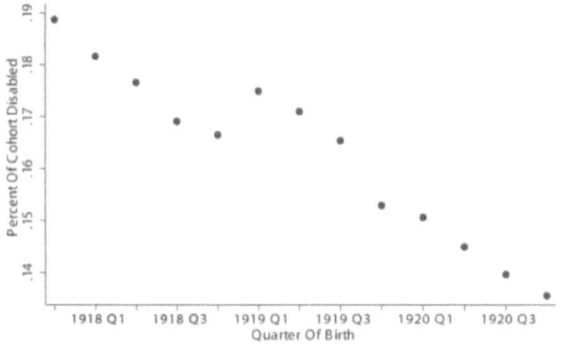

FIG. 2.—1980 male disability rates by quarter of birth: prevented from work by a physical disability.

Almond finds consequences many decades after the exposure. Health is found to affect every outcome. Women and men reveal discontinuous and big discounts in attainment when they'd been through the pandemic in utero. The children of infected mothers were up to 15 percent less likely to graduate from high school. Wages of men were reduced 9 percent due to disease. Socioeconomic status was considerably reduced, and the chance of being poor climbed up to 15 percent contrasted with different cohorts. Entitlement spending has been raised. At appropriate, as an instance, are male handicap rates in 1980, i.e. for men around age 60, by quarter and year of birth. Cohorts born between January and September of 1919 "were in utero in the height of this pandemic and are estimated to get 20 percent greater disability rates at age 61." Figure 3 to right reveals average years of education in 1960; once more the decrease is apparent for people born in 1918. Notice that not all pregnant women contracted flu, so the real effects of flu exposure are bigger, about a 5-month decrease in schooling, largely coming through reduced graduate prices. Education that is reduced and disability translate into government obligations

261

as revealed in the figure below. Almond labels these welfare payments, which might be slightly misleading. These are Social Security Disability payments in 1970. Here Is Almond:

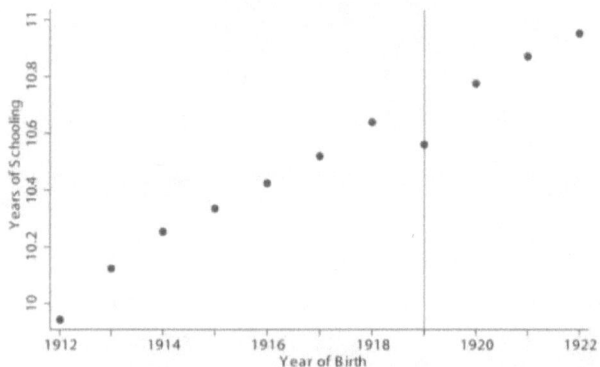

Fig. 3.—1960 average years of schooling: men and women born in the United States

Payments to nonwhites and women in 1970 are plotted in figure 8. The welfare payment was roughly one-third greater for children, or 12 percent greater for girls and nonwhites born in 1919. It's evident that premiums generate these payments to people when we concentrate on the quarter of birth.

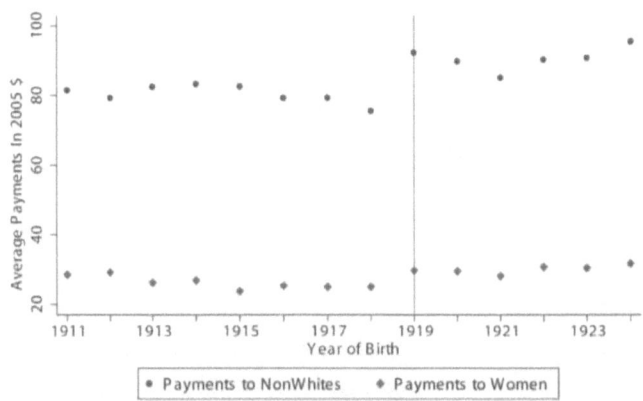

FIG. 8.—Average welfare payments for women and nonwhites: by year of birth

Notice that men and women that were disabled could have dead before 1970, and so these are lower bounds on the disability impact. The 1918 kids, for example, seem about the same as the 1920 kids, so it's not that the flu killed off the weak kids in 1918. Almond was interested in the 1918 pandemic not simply as a historical episode, but to make the case that infant health and infant health programs have a high benefit to cost ratios -- a still relevant lesson.

Chapter - 8 The 1918-19 Vaccine Development And Spanish Influenza Pandemic

When Individuals write about the Spanish Influenza outbreak of 1918-19, they begin with the death toll, the amount of inability of the area, and also individuals that have been infected with the virus. And while those variables were hallmarks of this catastrophic incident, researchers and health workers in the USA and Europe were devising vaccines and immunizing thousands and thousands of individuals in what amounted to medical experimentation on the greatest scale. What exactly were they with? Can they do anything to stop the spread of this illness and to safeguard the immunized? First, in 1918, the US population was 103.2 million. Throughout the 3 waves of the Spanish Influenza outbreak involving spring 1918 and spring 1919, roughly 200 of each 1000 people contracted flu (roughly 20.6 million). Between 0.8 percent (164,800) and 3.1 percent (638,000) of the infected died from flu or pneumonia secondary to it. A couple of vaccines to prevent different diseases were offered at that time-- smallpox vaccine had been utilized for over a hundred years; Louis Pasteur had developed rabies vaccine for post-exposure prophylaxis following an encounter with a rabid animal; typhoid fever vaccines were developed. Diphtheria antitoxin -- a medicine made from infected animals' bloodstream -- was used in the late 1800s for therapy; an early type of diphtheria vaccine was utilized, and cholera vaccines were developed. Almroth Wright had analyzed a vaccine in South African gold miners. Producers marketed and had developed different mixed inventory vaccines of usefulness. At the time, there wasn't a fantastic deal known concerning the understanding of flu as an infectious disease. Medical professionals believed that flu was a communicable disease that was introduced primarily in the winter. Without tools that are specific, cases of flu were hard to differentiate from respiratory disorders. They were able to discover germs, not pathogens.

And scientists and doctors struggled to know whether the annual flu to which they had been used was associated with the prevalent and thoroughly outbreak illness of decades we know was the pandemic flu (1848-49 and 1889-90). German scientist Richard Pfeiffer (1858-1945) claimed to have identified the causative agent of flu in a novel in 1892 -- he also explained rod-shaped bacilli within each event of flu he analyzed. He was able to demonstrate Koch's postulates by inducing the disease in experimental animals. Many specialists accepted his findings and believed Pfeiffer's influenza bacillus because it was accountable for seasonal flu. However, since methods improved, other investigators presented results that conflicted with the findings of Pfeiffer. They discovered his organism in healthy people and people suffering. They looked for Pfeiffer's bacillus in many cases and flu cases, but didn't find it. Though many doctors still thought that Pfeiffer had properly identified the offender, a rising number of others had started to doubt that his findings. Those true believers had any reason to be optimistic that a vaccine might protect against flu as the disease started its next appearance in the USA in early autumn 1918. From October 2, 1918, William H. Park, MD, mind bacteriologist of this New York City Health Department, was operating on a Pfeiffer's germs influenza vaccine. The New York Times reported that Royal S. Copeland, Health Commissioner of New York City, explained the vaccine like a flu preventative and also an "application of an old idea to a new disease." Park was building his vaccine out of heat-killed Pfeiffer's bacilli isolated from sick people and analyzing it on volunteers from Health Department personnel (New York Times, October 2, 1918). Three doses had been given 48 hours. From October 12, he wrote at the New York Medical Journal that he had been vaccinating workers from big businesses and soldiers in military camps. He expected to have proof to demonstrate the efficacy of the vaccine in a couple of months (Park WH, 1918).

In November, the Newark Evening News reported that 39,000 Doses of Leary-Park flu vaccine was prepared and doses had been used. (Timothy Leary was a professor at Tufts University School of Medicine.) Even though it was too soon to tell whether the vaccine was successful,". . . the average individual need not have any fear of the vaccine's outcomes. Neurotic and rheumatic people, nevertheless, seem to be more sensitive to the vaccine, while kids accept it with less interference than adults" (Newark Evening News, 1918). From December 13, 1918, Copeland wasn't so convinced about his section vaccine. He told the Times that vaccines produced from the bacilli of Pfeiffer seemed to have no impact on flu prevention. Instead, he was convinced that a combined bacterial vaccine (streptococcal, pneumococcal, staphylococcal, and Pfeiffer's bacilli) developed by E.C. Rosenow in the Mayo Foundation was a powerful preventative. And while he believed that many individuals in New York had been subjected to Spanish flu, he said he could have Park prepare a number of their Rosenow vaccines to

266

immunize individuals in New York through winter (New York Times, December 13, 1918). Well over 500,000 doses of Rosenow vaccine were created (Eyler, 2009).Tulane University, University of Pittsburgh, as well as personal doctors, were creating their vaccines. Convalescent serum was also utilized (Boston Post, January 6, 1919; Robertson & Koehler, 1918). The Deseret (UT) Evening News mentioned on December 14, 1918, that free vaccine was first available in communities across the nation. According to my survey of paper and recent clinical journal articles, it's apparent that lots of hundreds of thousands, maybe even a thousand or even more, doses of vaccines have been generated during the pandemic decades. (A couple of years back I wrote another blog article about Rosenow's vaccine) The Editorial Committee of the American Journal of Public Health attempted to place a damper on people's expectations concerning the vaccines. They composed in January 1919 the causative organism of this present influenza was unknown, and so the vaccines being generated had just an opportunity in being targeted at the ideal target. They noticed that vaccines for secondary ailments made a sense, but all the vaccines being generated have to be seen as experimental. Acknowledging the somewhat ad hoc character vaccine development from the present crisis, they advocated that management classes be utilized with the vaccines, which the differences between experimental and control group be lessened, as to the threat of exposure, time of exposure during the outbreak, etc (Editorial Committee of the American Journal of Public Health, 1919).

Surely none of the vaccines' viral flu infection -- we understand today that flu is brought on by a virus, and not one of the vaccines protected against it. But were any of these

267

protective from the bacterial diseases that developed secondary to flu? Vaccinologist Stanley A. Plotkin, MD, believes that they weren't. He advised us: "The bacterial vaccines designed for Spanish flu were probably ineffective since at the time it wasn't understood that pneumococcal bacteria come in many, several serotypes and of their bacterial group they predicted B. influenza, just 1 form is a significant pathogen." To put it differently, the vaccine programmers had little capability to identify, isolate, and create all of the possible disease-causing strains of germs circulating at the moment. Now there's a pneumococcal vaccine for kids that protects against 13 serotypes of the germs, along with the vaccine for adults shields against 23 serotypes. A 2010 informative article, however, describes a meta-analysis of bacterial vaccine research from 1918-19 and indicates a more positive interpretation. According to the 13 studies that met inclusion criteria, the authors conclude that a few of the vaccines might have decreased the assault speed of pneumonia following viral flu infection. They imply that regardless of the restricted quantities of bacteria strains from the vaccines, vaccination might have resulted in cross-protection from multiple associated breeds (Chien, 2010). It wasn't until the 1930s that investigators established that the flu was brought on by a virus, not a bacterium. Pfeiffer's flu bacillus would finally be termed Haemophilus influenzae, the title keeping the heritage of its longstanding, though incorrect, association with flu. And now, flu vaccines -- also as H. influenzae type b vaccines – are broadly available to reduce disease.

Influenza Vaccine

Influenza vaccines, also known as flu shots or influenza jabs, are compounds that protect against infection by influenza viruses. New variations of these vaccines have been developed twice annually since the flu virus immediately changes. Even though their effectiveness varies from year to year, many supply modest to high security against flu. The United States Centers for Disease Control and Prevention (CDC) estimates that vaccination against flu reduces illness, clinical visits, hospitalizations, and deaths. Immunized employees, who do catch the flu, come back to work half a day earlier on average. Vaccine efficacy in people under two years old and people over 65 years old remains unclear because of a shortage of high excellent research. Vaccinating kids can protect those around them.

The World Health Organization (WHO) and the U.S. Centers for Disease Control and Prevention (CDC) recommend yearly vaccination for almost all people over age six months, particularly those at high risk. The European Centre for Disease Prevention and Control (ECDC) additionally urges annual vaccination for these high-risk groups: pregnant women, the elderly, and children between six months and five decades old, those with specific health issues, and people who are employed in health care.

The vaccines are safe. Fever occurs in five to ten percent of children vaccinated. Muscle aches or feelings of fatigue may occur. At a speed of approximately one case per million doses, the vaccine was associated with a rise in Guillain syndrome among individuals in certain years. They are suggested that flu vaccines are generated using eggs. Influenza vaccines aren't recommended in those who've experienced a serious allergy to versions of the vaccine. The vaccine comes from diminished forms that are viral and dormant. The weakened vaccine in individuals with a weakened immune system, children, adults, or recommended in pregnant women. Based upon the kind they are sometimes injected into a muscle, then sprayed into the nose, or inserted into the center of skin (intradermal). The vaccine wasn't available throughout 2018-2019 and 2019-2020 flu seasons. Vaccination against the flu started in the 1930s. It's about the List of Essential Medicines, the most powerful and best medicines of the World Health Organization. The wholesale cost in the developing world is roughly US $5.25 per dose as of 2014. In the USA, the vaccine prices less than US$25 as part of 2015, each dose.

Medical Uses

The U.S Centers for Disease Control and Prevention (CDC) urges the flu vaccine in order to stop its spread and protect individuals. When someone buys, anxiety that the vaccine didn't contain the influenza vaccine may decrease the severity of influenza. It requires about two weeks after vaccination for antibodies that are protective to form. A 2012 meta-analysis discovered that influenza vaccination was successful 67 percent of their time; the inhabitants that benefited the most were HIV-positive adults aged 18 to 55 (76 percent), healthy adults aged 18 to 46 (roughly 70 percent), and wholesome children aged six to 24 months (66 percent). The flu vaccine also seems to protect against myocardial infarction using a benefit of 15 to 45 percent.

Effectiveness

There is a vaccine evaluated by its effectiveness -- the extent to which It reduces its efficacy -- the reduction in risk after the vaccine is put into use -- and also a risk of disorder under controlled conditions. In the event of flu, since it's quantified utilizing the degrees efficacy it is forecasted to be lower. Influenza vaccines show efficacy. Yet, studies on the efficacy of influenza vaccines in the actual world are hard; vaccines could be imperfectly coordinated, virus incidence varies widely between years, and flu can be confused with other influenza-like ailments. But in most years (16 of those 19 years earlier 2007), the influenza vaccine strains are a fantastic match for its circulating strains, and even a mismatched vaccine could frequently offer cross-protection. The virus varies due to drift, a mutation in the virus which is responsible for a breed. Yearly influenza vaccination that is repeated offers you constant protection against flu. There's indicative evidence that repeated vaccinations might make a decrease in vaccine efficacy for specific flu subtypes; this does not have any significance to present recommendations for annual vaccinations but may influence future vaccination coverage. As of 2019, a vaccine is recommended by the CDC since studies reveal the efficacy of influenza vaccination.

Criticism

Influenza vaccines have predicted clinical signs concerning influenza vaccines "rap" and has consequently declared them to be unsuccessful; it's known for esophageal clinical trials, which many in the area maintain as unethical. Institutions such as the CDC and the National Institutes of Health, also from key figures in the area such as Anthony Fauci reject his perspectives on the effectiveness of influenza vaccines. Michael Osterholm, who headed the Center for Infectious Disease Research and Policy 2012 review on influenza vaccines, advocated getting the vaccine but criticized its promotion, stating, "We've over-promoted and overhyped this particular vaccine... it doesn't shield as encouraged. It is a sales job: it is all public relations."

Kids

The CDC recommends that everybody except babies under the age of six months must get the seasonal flu vaccine. Vaccination campaigns generally focus particular attention on individuals that are at elevated risk of severe complications if they catch the flu, such as elderly women, kids under 59 weeks, the elderly, and individuals with chronic illnesses or weakened immune systems, in addition to individuals to whom they are vulnerable, such as healthcare workers. Since the departure rate is too high among babies who catch flu, the CDC and the WHO recommend that household contacts and caregivers of babies be vaccinated to decrease the danger of passing a flu infection to the baby. In children, the vaccine seems to lower the chance of potential disease and flu. In children under the age of 2, information is constrained. Throughout 2017-18 flu season, the CDC manager suggested that 85 percent of those kids who died "probably weren't vaccinated." In the USA, in January 2019, the CDC recommends that children aged six through 35 months can receive either 0.25 milliliters or 0.5 milliliters per dose of Fluzone Quadrivalent. There's not any preference for one of the dose quantity of Fluzone Quadrivalent for this age category. All men 36 weeks of age and older must get 0.5 milliliters per dose of Fluzone Quadrivalent. In October 2018, Afluria Quadrivalent is accredited for children six months old and older from the United States Children six months through 35 months old should get 0.25 milliliters for every dose of Afluria

Quadrivalent. All men 36 weeks of age and older must get 0.5 milliliters per dose of Afluria Quadrivalent. As of February 2018, Afluria Tetra is accredited for children and adults five decades old and older in Canada. In 2014, the Canadian National Advisory Committee on Immunization (NACI) released an overview of flu vaccination in healthy 5-18-year-olds, also in 2015, printed a report on using pediatric Fluad in kids 6-72 weeks old.

16 percent get symptoms like the flu, adults, while about 10 percent of adults do. Vaccination decreased confirmed cases of flu from roughly 2.4 percent to 1.1 percent. No impact on the operation was discovered. In adults, a review from the Cochrane Collaboration found without impacting transmission or influenza-related complications that hepatitis led to days lost and a reduction in both flu symptoms. In healthy functioning adults, flu vaccines may offer mild protection from virologically- confirmed influenza, although such defense is significantly diminished or absent in certain seasons. In healthcare employees, a benefit was discovered by a 2006 evaluation. Of the studies in this review, just two also evaluated the relationship of individual mortality relative to employees flu vaccine uptake; equally discovered that greater rates of healthcare employee vaccination associated with decreased patient deaths. A 2014 review found advantages to patients when healthcare employees were immunized, as encouraged by moderate signs predicated in part on the observed reduction in all-cause deaths in patients that their healthcare employees were granted immunization compared in comparison to patients in which the employees weren't provided disease.

273

Mature

Evidence for an effect in adults more than 65 years old is unclear. Systematic reviews analyzing the case and controlled, control studies found that a deficiency of signs that is high quality. Reviews of the case-control studies found effects against flu, pneumonia, and death. The older, the group most vulnerable to flu, benefits from the embryo. There are reasons for this decrease in vaccine efficiency, the most frequent of which would be associated with age and the immunological role. In a non-pandemic calendar year, an individual in the USA aged 50-64 is almost ten times more likely to die an influenza-associated departure than a younger man, and a man over age 65 is more than ten times more likely to die an influenza-associated departure compared to 50-64 age category. An influenza vaccine is formulated to offer a more powerful immune reaction. Evidence suggests that vaccinating the elderly leads to the vaccine. An influenza vaccine comprising an adjuvant was accepted by the U.S. Food and Drug Administration (FDA) in November 2015, to be used by adults aged 65 decades old and older. The vaccine is promoted as Fluad from the U.S. and was available in the 2016-2017 flu period. The vaccine includes the MF59C.1 adjuvant that is an oil-in-water emulsion of squalene oil. It's the seasonal influenza vaccine. It isn't clear if there's a substantial advantage for the elderly to utilize an influenza vaccine comprising the MF59C.1 adjuvant. Fluad may be utilized as an alternate approved for individuals 65 decades and older. It is advocated to decrease flu outbreaks in these people. Even though there's absolutely no evidence from trials that healthcare employees help protect older people, there is evidence of advantage.

Chapter - 9 Lessons In The 1918 Spanish Flu Pandemic

MONDAY, April 20, 2020 (Health Day News) -- "The virus struck dread since it murdered tens of thousands and sickened millions -- and today the 1918 influenza pandemic provides courses. "The questions they asked then are the questions being asked today," explained Christopher Nichols, an associate professor of history at Oregon State University, in Corvallis. "And while it is very rare that background gives a simple straightforward lesson to the current, this is one of these cases." Experts say that there are four important takeaways in 1918.

Here is the first:

"As devastating as the present pandemic could be, the Spanish influenza pandemic is still the worst in history," said E. Thomas Ewing, a history professor at Virginia Tech in Blacksburg. From now three waves of influenza swept across the world at least 50 million people have been dead. In contrast, influenza pandemics in 1957, 1968, and 2009 maintained an estimated total of 225,000 Americans and 3 million individuals worldwide.)

Here is the 2nd:

There are differences between the COVID-19 and 1918 pandemic. "Afterward they did not even know that it was a virus," Ewing said. "There'd been years of research about microbes, so that they knew that it had been moved person-to-person through respiratory drops, by coughing and sneezing. But viruses were not found until the 1930s since they did not have strong enough microscopes." Because of this, testing was difficult to find. It did not exist. Influenza-caused disorders were more infectious than COVID-19 and were much more deadly, Nichols explained. And that presents the best threat to older influenza. "It influenced everyone old and young," Nichols explained. "However, it killed the safest one of people: an all-American 22-year-old soccer player. Individuals in their prime got struck down. So, the panic that animated men and women in the autumn of 1918 were different."

Here is the 3rd:

Despite these differences, 2020 is striking. There was no cure for the disease and no vaccine a healthcare system might decode. And here is takeaway No. 4: In both pandemics, the best immediate response was -- and is social distancing, Nichols explained. "It was known as crowding' control back then," he explained. "However, whatever you call it, restricting contact functioned in 1918 -- and it functions now." Along with distancing and the comprehensive closures are set into position, the faster a pandemic could be brought under control, Nichols added. People who lived through influenza discovered that lesson the hard way, based on Carolyn Orban in Columbia.

"Like pandemics, in 1918 you had stress between biological

truth and socioeconomic fact," she explained. "Biology isn't changeable. But behavior is. Yes, social distancing was a thing in 1918, also in which it had been practiced, it worked."

However mistrust, from fear, fear interests -- and even boredom many were fast to jump ship and slow to have on board. Historians see the signs in letters written in precisely the time by the families. "The mom is saying, 'We all must be patient, lay low and wait it out,' while the kid is saying she has had enough of no faculty and no friends, and she is planning a Halloween celebration, in the same way, the maximum amount of deaths are occurring," Orban clarified. That tension helps clarify the lack of a strong and ancient reaction according to Ewing and Nichols. Officials stalled for a while and played down the danger. Why? Some motives were exceptional to 1918. "The hay strike throughout a critical phase of World War I," Nichols explained. "From the time the initial presumed U.S. instance was identified in March 1918 in a Kansas army foundation, there was great concern about soldiers becoming ill. That issue was well-founded: Army camps' quarters were dishes for sickness," Orban explained.

"Boys will... return in body bags in these amounts that finally it became nearly impossible to distinguish the war effort from the pandemic," she explained. And early on, the authorities had the reason Nichols mentioned. Flu deaths were reduced and tens of thousands of troops were led into the front lines in Europe. "The focus is completely on the last major push to finish the war," he clarified. So, the information from Washington, D.C., back then may seem familiar now: Do not panic. It is no big thing. "Initially they inform the public it is not a large issue, or even -- as its name implies -- that it is a foreign disorder that only affects 'other people.'

Conclusion

Nichols said, "It was not until the autumn, following a more virulent type of Spanish influenza had emerged, that Washington, D.C., obtained rough. Meanwhile, the lack of a federal reaction left states and cities to go off by themselves and make decisions for them." Nichols said the market was chosen by many plus distancing is placing off by them, together with outcomes. Many others didn't while cities such as Seattle and San Francisco ordered people to wear masks when they had been out in public. Colleges never shut, asserting that they were cleaner. Many cities failed, although October 1918, when deaths started to skyrocket. According to Ewing, "There were lots of inconsistencies." Two studies published at the Proceedings of the National Academy of Sciences in 2007 looked at the impact of health measures, such as business-hour limitations, mask legislation, along with the shuttering of dancing halls and colleges, theaters, and churches in over 15 cities in 1918. Both studies found that towns which acted most forcefully -- such as St. Louis, that imposed a near-complete lockdown in two weeks of its initial Spanish influenza instance -- had considerably lower summit departure rates than towns which hedged their bets -- such as New Orleans, Boston, and Philadelphia. The point isn't so social networking is a complete panacea, but there's no "business-as-usual throughout a pandemic," Nichols explained.

So the lesson of 1918 is apparent: "If people's wellness is the principal focus, then eliminate that from your head," Nichols said. "Spanish influenza informs us that social networking works. It works best when we act and adhere together -- and

279

base our conclusions not on social or financial issues, but data, science, and details.